Practical Management of Dementia: a multi-professional approach

Edited by

Stephen Curran

Consultant and Visiting Professor of Old Age Psychopharmacology
School of Human and Health Sciences
University of Huddersfield

and

John P Wattis

Consultant and Visiting Professor of Old Age Psychiatry
School of Human and Health Sciences
University of Huddersfield

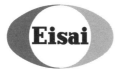 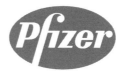

Provided by way of an educational grant as a service to medicine by Eisai Limited & Pfizer Limited.
The opinions of the authors in this publication may or may not reflect those of Eisai/Pfizer.
Eisai/Pfizer accepts no liability for opinions or statements made by any authors.

RADCLIFFE MEDICAL PRESS
OXFORD • SAN FRANCISCO

Radcliffe Medical Press Ltd
18 Marcham Road
Abingdon
Oxon OX14 1AA
United Kingdom

www.radcliffe-oxford.com
The Radcliffe Medical Press electronic catalogue and online ordering facility.
Direct sales to anywhere in the world.

British Library Cataloguing in Publication Data

A catalogue record for this book is available from the British Library.

ISBN 1 85775 931 1

Typeset by Acorn Bookwork Ltd, Salisbury
Printed and bound by TJ International Ltd, Padstow, Cornwall

Contents

Preface

In this book we have brought together findings from recent research with a multidisciplinary perspective into the practical aspects of dementia care. We strongly believe in the importance of bringing together the best in research and practice. When these are divorced, researchers may lose the vision of the real purpose of their work and practitioners may not have access to the most recent advances in knowledge. We hope this book will help bridge that gap. We have chosen our contributors mostly for their knowledge and practical experience in their own fields but also because of their expertise in policy and teaching. Looking after the needs of people with dementia demands a multi-talented, multidisciplinary approach. Practice in this field needs to be rooted in respect for the personhood of people with dementia. It needs to be underpinned by political support. Organisations like the Alzheimer's Society perform an invaluable function in campaigning on behalf of patients and their relatives. Nevertheless, issues like the closure of residential and nursing homes for largely financial reasons, despite the impact on residents, many of whom suffer from dementia, continue to cause concern.

If we ever develop dementia, we would like people to notice it early. We would like them to respect our autonomy but steer us quickly in the direction of the best help available. We would like to be seen by appropriately qualified people who could make a diagnosis and provide any useful medical treatment, social, psychological, nursing and therapy support and advice to ourselves and our families, and a truly personal approach to our needs, especially our spiritual needs. We hope this book will help people in developing the kind of services we would like to receive!

Stephen Curran
John Wattis
January 2004

About the editors

Stephen Curran works as a Consultant Old Age Psychiatrist in Wakefield, and has recently been appointed a Visiting Professor at Huddersfield University. He graduated in psychology before studying medicine and then worked as a Research Fellow and Lecturer in Old Age Psychiatry at the University of Leeds. His research interest is in psychopharmacology in older people with mental illness, particularly the pharmacological management of depression and early detection of Alzheimer's disease. He has numerous research publications to his credit, and has co-authored or co-edited a number of books.

John Wattis was appointed Visiting Professor of Psychiatry for Older Adults at Huddersfield University in 2000. Before this he was responsible for pioneering old age services in Leeds, where he worked as a Consultant and Senior Lecturer for nearly 20 years. He completed his psychiatric training in Birmingham and Nottingham, where he was a lecturer in the Department of Health Care of the Elderly, which combined psychiatric and medical teams. He has management experience as Medical Director of a large community and mental health trust. He is a former Chairman of the Faculty for Psychiatry of Old Age at the Royal College of Psychiatrists, and of the committee that advises on the higher training of doctors in general and old age psychiatry. He has published research on the development of old age psychiatry services, alcohol abuse in old age, the prevalence of mental illness in geriatric medical patients, and outcomes of psychiatric admission for older people. He has written or edited a number of books and contributed numerous chapters in the area of old age psychiatry.

Together, Stephen and John have contributed to undergraduate and postgraduate teaching both of doctors and of those in other disciplines. Their approach to healthcare for older people is founded on three principles:

1 recognition of the importance of *good relationships* between individuals and between different health and social care providers

2 firm commitment to the need to *develop and integrate evidence-based practice*

3 an emphasis on the need for *creativity in improving treatment and services.*

They are committed to a multidisciplinary and inter-agency approach to healthcare of the elderly that sees mental health and illness in the context of physical health and social pressures.

About the contributors

Dorrie Ball, Senior Lecturer in Social Work/Health and Social Care, School of Human and Health Sciences, University of Huddersfield

Peter Bowie, Senior Lecturer in Old Age Psychiatry, Academic Unit of Psychiatry and Behavioural Sciences, University of Leeds

Roger Bullock, Consultant in Old Age Psychiatry, Kingshill Research Centre, Victoria Hospital, Swindon

Michael A Carpenter, Consultant Physician, Medical Rehabilitation Unit, Pinderfields General Hospital, Wakefield

Richard J Clibbens, Nurse Consultant in Older People's Mental Health, South West Yorkshire Mental Health NHS Trust, Fieldhead Hospital, Wakefield

Stephen Curran, Consultant and Visiting Professor of Old Age Psychopharmacology, School of Human and Health Sciences, University of Huddersfield

Tony Dearden, Consultant in Old Age Psychiatry, Aire Court Community Unit, Leeds and Associate Medical Director, Leeds Mental Health Teaching NHS Trust

Mary Duggan, Strategic Planning Manager, South West Yorkshire Mental Health NHS Trust, Aberford Centre, Wakefield

Andrew M Ellis, Consultant Psychiatrist, Older People's Mental Health Services, Department of Psychiatry, Clatterbridge Hospital, Bebington, Wirral

Nick Farrar, Service Co-ordination Manager, Bradford Social Services

Linda Harris, General Practitioner, Homestead Clinic, Wakefield

Dianne Lewis MBE., Nurse Consultant in Care of Older People, Calderdale and Huddersfield NHS Trust, Huddersfield

Ann McPherson, Project Manager – Mental Health Out of Area Placements, South West Yorkshire Mental Health NHS Trust, Fieldhead, Wakefield

Edgar Miller, Professor of Psychology, University of Leicester

Shabir Musa, Consultant in Old Age Psychiatry, South West Yorkshire Mental Health NHS Trust, Chantry Unit, Fieldhead Hospital, Wakefield

Anna V Richman, Specialist Registrar in Old Age Psychiatry, Academic Unit, Elderly Mental Health Directorate, St Catherine's Hospital, Birkenhead

Loopinder Sood, Staff Grade Psychiatrist, South Warwickshire Assertive Outreach Team, St Michael's Hospital, Warwick

Yahya Takriti, Specialist Registrar in Old Age Psychiatry, South West Yorkshire Mental Health NHS Trust, Fieldhead, Wakefield

Daphne Wallace, Former Consultant in Old Age Psychiatry, Leeds and Wharfdale Psychology and Psychotherapy Practice, Otley

John P Wattis, Consultant and Visiting Professor of Old Age Psychiatry, School of Human and Health Sciences, University of Huddersfield

Ken CM Wilson, Professor of Old Age Psychiatry, Academic Unit, Elderly Mental Health Directorate, St Catherine's Hospital, Birkenhead

Acknowledgements

The editors would like to thank Patricia Robinson, Medical Secretary, Fieldhead Hospital, Wakefield for all her help and support with the many administrative tasks associated with the preparation of this book.

1
Dementia in the new millennium

John P Wattis

A brief history of our understanding of dementia

Like other mental illnesses, dementia bears a stigma. Before effective pharmacological measures for mental illness were developed, that is, before the last half of the twentieth century, different models for understanding mental illness and different modes of treatment prevailed. The first positive post-medieval development was that of 'moral management' or 'moral treatment' of mental illness. Previously, belief in demonology or views on the irrationality of people with mental illness had led to abuse and/or containment. Moral management brought about an engagement with the mentally ill person on an individual and collective level, reflected in the modern Therapeutic Community movement. Reasoning and moral and emotional support produced good results in places like the Retreat in York, England and in other countries too. The era of the large asylum and 'medicalisation' of mental illness followed. At the same time, the new discipline of psychoanalysis provided an explanation and treatment for some of the less severe mental disorders and had a wide impact on society. Critiques of an excessively medical model for understanding dementia[1] have led to practical measures for the well-being of patients with dementia[2] and recommendations for improved models of care.[3]

Although conditions described in Roman times probably correspond to current diagnoses of dementia, the modern *medical* history of the condition begins in 1906 when Alzheimer, a German neuropsychiatrist and associate of Kraeplin, described a woman in late middle age with the clinical picture and pathology of the disease that now bears his name. At another time, he also described the pathology of vascular dementia. At the time most cases of dementia in old people were written off as 'senile' dementia or 'senility'. Competing schools of neuropathology in Munich (Alzheimer) and Prague perpetuated this divide and the identity of Alzheimer's disease in most cases of 'senile' dementia was not widely realised for another half century.

In the mid-1950s, Roth[4] published an account of the natural history of mental disorders in old age that distinguished between 'senile' and 'arteriosclerotic' psychoses on the basis of their outcomes. Further studies established the epidemiology of mental disorders in late life[5] and the quantitative pathology[6] of Alzheimer's and vascular dementia. The deficiency of the neurotransmitter, acetylcholine, in Alzheimer's disease was recognised ten years later[7] and led to the development of the cholinergic hypothesis and therapies based upon it. Initially these were based upon attempts to increase the availability of choline by dietary supplementation with the precursor lecithin, and subsequently on inhibition of the enzymes responsible for breaking down acetylcholine. In the meantime, specialist mental health services for older people were developing and taking an interest in the positive management of people with dementia.[8] At this time Alzheimer's and vascular dementia were regarded as the two main causes of dementia, accounting singly or in combination for 90% or more of all cases (see Chapter 2). There were a host of other rarer causes, such as Pick's disease and the 'metabolic' dementias of vitamin B_{12} and thyroid deficiency (see Chapter 7). More recently, diffuse Lewy body dementia has been recognised,[9] though it has still not been included in international diagnostic systems and there is still debate about its precise relationship with Alzheimer's disease, Parkinson's disease and other psychiatric disorders.[10,11] Often different types of pathology co-exist. The 'nun study' showed the importance of vascular damage in producing clinical dementia in patients with co-existing Alzheimer pathology,[12] confirming earlier pathological studies.

The burden of dementia

Dementia imposes a terrible burden on society. The social burden is greatly influenced by demography since dementia is predominantly a condition of very old people. Since the beginning of the twentieth century, the proportion of people in the United Kingdom (UK) over the age of 65 has risen threefold. The proportion of very old has increased even more markedly. Other countries in the developed world have been through similar changes, and these changes are likely to be experienced in an accelerated way in the developing world (see Chapter 2).

Society may also increase the personal burden on people with dementia and those who care for them by the way it reacts to people with dementia (see Chapter 11) and by placing them and their carers under economic pressure. Political decisions about eligibility for care services supported by the State affect the financial burden. There is need for a debate about why old people with dementia should receive less favourable social support than young people with physical disability. For individuals afflicted with dementia, the eventual loss of capacity for independent living threatens to take away their autonomy. For family and other carers there is the constant worry about safety and the burden of directly or indirectly meeting the needs of those who find it increasingly difficult to care for themselves. In the UK, around three-quarters of a million people are currently affected.[13] In the United States (US), the comparable figure is around four million.[14] Currently, between 18 and 37 million people worldwide are estimated to have one or other type of dementia and projections suggest that by 2025 this number will nearly double, with nearly three-quarters living in developing countries (see Chapter 2). The cost in terms of lost human potential and burden on care-givers is vast; current annual costs in the US alone are estimated at over $100 billion. Despite the fact that dementia is concentrated in late life, it ranks

13th in the World Health Organization's (WHO) list of causes of years lived with disability.[15] What can be done about so great a burden?

What we can do

We need to respond to the challenge at a variety of levels, including:

- the international level
- the national level
- the level of the local community
- the level of the family
- the personal level.

Internationally, organisations like Alzheimer's International, WHO and the International Psychogeriatric Association are trying to prepare countries in the developing world for the explosion in the prevalence of dementia that an ageing population will bring. In the developed world, there is still a need to eradicate ageist attitudes to the provision of support and treatment for people with dementia. At the population level, our developing knowledge of the risk factors for various forms of dementia may well enable us to produce a relative reduction in the numbers of people affected. However, *age itself* is the greatest risk factor for developing dementia, especially Alzheimer's disease, and so all those public health and lifestyle measures that increase longevity are likely to increase the population at risk. This does not mean we should give up. Reducing the prevalence of disease and its impact are fundamental tasks for medicine, related disciplines and the whole of society.

The 'ideal' scenario would be to develop the capacity to identify people at risk of dementia and to reduce that risk by acceptable and inexpensive public health or specific treatment measures. Genetic risk factors are already identified and will be discussed in more detail in Chapters 2 and 3. Measures to eliminate these genes from the gene pool are likely to be impractical, morally unacceptable and have unforeseeable consequences. However, genotyping to identify 'at risk' populations may, as our knowledge of the mechanisms of disease expands, enable preventive measures or early treatment at a pre-clinical stage before symptoms of disease develop. As new drugs are developed that interfere with the progression of Alzheimer's disease, and as the population of the developing world ages, dilemmas are likely to occur about the affordability of these drugs in poorer countries. Local communities need to be helped to develop a better understanding of dementia and the issues that surround it so that families and people with dementia are treated as people and not marginalised. Old age psychiatry services, working through local government and primary care services, should see this education as one of their functions.

At the family and individual level, positive management requires a biopsycho-

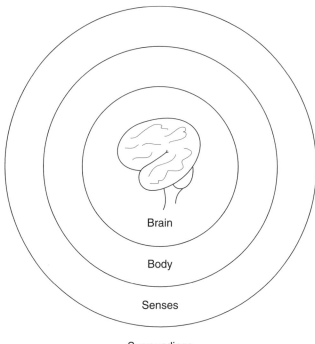

Brain

Body

Senses

Surroundings

Figure 1.1   An interactive model of confusion.[16]

social model. A model that only considers one of these factors is wholly inadequate. Figure 1.1 emphasises that in dealing with any individual patient, we
need to take into account brain, body, senses and physical and social environment *and the interaction between them*.[16]

Positive management of dementia consists of first making a diagnosis and
excluding rare, potentially treatable causes of dementia such as thyroid deficiency. Specific treatment for Alzheimer's dementia now exists and is probably
effective in some other forms of dementia too, though use of the drugs in some
countries is constrained by government guidelines.[17] The next step is to maximise
the patient's capacity for independent living by optimising physical health,
correcting deficiencies in hearing and sight and providing a supportive environment. Emotional and practical support to patients and carers requires collaboration across health and social care organisations. This kind of multi-layered
approach was fostered and strengthened by the multidisciplinary approach to
old age mental health services developed in the UK.[18–20] Other interventions,
psychological and pharmacological, are required to cope with the depression and
behavioural problems sometimes found in people with dementia.

However, even in the UK, one of the first countries to develop specific old age
psychiatry services, there is a 'clinical iceberg'. The majority of people with
dementia never come to the attention of those specialist services. There is a major
need for specialist services to work together with primary care to improve access

to those specialist services for people with dementia. The arrival of drugs for the treatment of Alzheimer's disease has increased the number of referrals and, in the UK, specialist memory clinics are increasing in number to cope with increased demand.[21]

Future directions

The first useful anti-dementia drugs, the cholinesterase inhibitors, have now been available for over five years. These drugs (tacrine, donepezil, rivastigmine, galantamine and others) interfere with the breakdown of acetylcholine, effectively amplifying its effect at the synaptic cleft. Memantine, a drug with a completely different mode of action, has also been licensed in the UK for moderate to severe dementia of the Alzheimer type. Other existing drugs, such as the non-steroidal anti-inflammatory drugs (NSAIDs), oestrogens and nicotine, may also have some effect on Alzheimer's dementia. It seems likely that anti-platelet drugs will help some patients with vascular dementia, though this has yet to be convincingly demonstrated. Drugs currently in development may affect the development of the insoluble form of beta-amyloid by inhibiting some of the enzymes that split amyloid precursor protein. Attempts to deal with amyloid by inducing an immune response have had to be abandoned because in clinical trials they appeared to induce an immune response to other parts of the central nervous system. Other lines of enquiry, especially into the genetic risk factors for Alzheimer's and other dementias, are likely to suggest further therapeutic avenues. The herbal preparation, Gingko biloba, has also been shown to have some positive effect in Alzheimer's disease, though the mechanism of action is not clear. If we did understand it better, perhaps this too would suggest other lines of approach.

However, the future does not only lie in developing new drugs. Basic science may help us understand the processes that precede the clinical symptoms of Alzheimer's disease and may suggest preventive measures we cannot anticipate. Psychological and social care for people with dementia will develop. Indeed, we could improve considerably on our current practical care for people with dementia by implementing what we already know and by educating those involved in providing care to people with dementia in the principles of person-centred care.[22] Improving the organisation and management of care should not be neglected either. This requires a more adequate political and social response to the challenges posed by an ageing society.

Practical management of dementia

The scope of what we currently can do is very wide and this book seeks to explore that scope. It does not look in detail at the anti-dementia drugs, though these are mentioned briefly in Chapter 12 'The role of the memory clinic'. We have asked contributors to cover epidemiology (the science of the distribution of disease in populations), and the current classification of the dementias into different diagnoses with different causes, time courses and (potentially) treatments. Building on that foundation, we have looked at the practical science of early detection and diagnosis. We have also taken a variety of perspectives: those of the psychiatrist, clinical psychologist, physician for the elderly, the general practitioner (GP), the nurse, the occupational therapist and the social worker. We have explored the role of the 'memory clinic' and the special issues of early-onset dementia. We have also asked contributors to discuss the legal framework in which we manage dementia (principally from the point of view of English law) and to share neglected but developing knowledge about the spiritual aspects of dementia and its management. Finally, we have commissioned a chapter to discuss how comprehensive and integrated mental health services for people with dementia might be developed, rooted largely in practice in the UK. As in any edited work we are conscious of some repetitions, but in an effort to make each chapter reasonably self-sufficient we have not tried to eliminate these.

We are in the middle of an exciting decade when major scientific advances in the diagnosis and management of Alzheimer's disease and other forms of dementia are likely to occur. These advances will require political commitment and financial support if they are to bear fruit in preventing[23] or delaying the onset of dementia and in improving the quality of life of people with dementia and those who care for them. In the meantime, this book aims to be a useful, practical guide to the current state of knowledge about the management of dementia. By approaching the problems of dementia from a multidisciplinary perspective, we hope to stimulate the creativity of our readers in developing and implementing best practice in dementia care.

Key points

- The modern 'biomedical' understanding of dementia is only a century old.
- It is inadequate without a broader 'psychosocial' approach.
- The burden on society from dementia is related to an ageing population.
- The burden on individuals with dementia and their carers is worsened by ageism manifested in reduced support when compared with chronic disabilities affecting younger people.
- International and national action is needed to meet the political and economic challenges of an ageing population and an increased prevalence of dementia.
- Local communities can respond with more understanding if old age services make education part of their task.
- Families and people with dementia can be helped by an integrated biological, psychological and social approach in a multidisciplinary framework.
- This book seeks to set out the current 'state of the art' of practical provision for people with dementia and aims to stimulate creative innovation.

References

1   Kitwood T (1990) The dialectics of dementia, with particular reference to Alzheimer's disease. *Ageing and Society.* **10**: 177–96.

2   Kitwood T and Bredin K (1992) A new approach to the evaluation of dementia care. *Journal of Advances in Health and Nursing Care.* **1**(5): 41–60.

3   Kitwood T (1997) *Dementia Reconsidered: the person comes first.* Open University Press, Buckingham.

4   Roth M (1955) The natural history of mental disorder in old age. *Journal of Mental Science.* **101**: 281–301.

5   Kay DW, Beamish P and Roth M (1964) Old age mental disorders in Newcastle-upon-Tyne. Part I: A study of prevalence. *British Journal of Psychiatry.* **110**: 146–58.

6   Blessed G, Tomlinson BE and Roth M (1968) The association between quantitative measures of dementia and senile change in the grey matter of elderly people. *British Journal of Psychiatry.* **144**: 797–811.

7   Perry E, Tomlinson BE, Bergmann K *et al.* (1978) Correlation of cholinergic abnormalities with senile plaques and mental test scores in senile dementia. *British Medical Journal.* **2**: 1457–9.

8   Arie T (1971) The morale and planning of psychogeriatric services. *British Medical Journal.* **iii**: 166–70.

9   Forstl H, Burns A, Luthert P *et al.* (1993) The Lewy body variant of Alzheimer's disease: clinical and pathological findings. *British Journal of Psychiatry.* **162**: 385–92.

10 Byrne EJ (1992) Diffuse Lewy body disease: spectrum disorder or variety of Alzheimer's disease? *International Journal of Geriatric Psychiatry.* **7**: 229–34.

11 Birkett P, Desouky A, Han L *et al.* (1992) Lewy bodies in psychiatric patients. *International Journal of Geriatric Psychiatry.* **7**: 235–40.

12 Snowdon DA, Greiner LH, Mortimer JA *et al.* (1997) Brain infarction and the clinical expression of Alzheimer disease. The Nun Study. *Journal of the American Medical Association.* **227**: 813–17.

13 Alzheimer's Society website (2002): www.alzheimers.org.uk/about/statistics. html

14 Alzheimer's Association website (2002): www.alz.org/hc/overview/stats.htm

15 World Health Organization (2001) *World Health Report 2001.* WHO, Geneva.

16 Wattis J and Curran S (2001) *The Practical Psychiatry of Old Age.* Radcliffe Medical Press, Oxford.

17 National Institute for Clinical Excellence (2001) *The Use of Donepezil, Rivastigmine and Galantamine in the Treatment of Alzheimer's Disease.* NICE, London.

18 Wattis JP, Wattis L and Arie TH (1981) Psychogeriatrics: a national survey of a new branch of psychiatry. *British Medical Journal.* **282**: 1529–33.

19 Wattis JP (1988) Geographical variations in the provision of psychiatric services for old people. *Age and Ageing.* **17**: 171–80.

20 Wattis J, Macdonald A and Newton P (1999) Old age psychiatry: a specialty in transition – results of the 1996 survey. *Psychiatric Bulletin.* **23**: 331–5.

21 Lindesay J, Marudkar M, van Diepen E *et al.* (2002) The second Leicester

survey of memory clinics in the British Isles. *International Journal of Geriatric Psychiatry*. **17**: 41–7.

22 Kitwood T and Bredin K (1992) *Person to Person: a guide to the care of those with failing mental powers*. Gale Centre Publications, Loughton.

23 Lautenschlager NT, Almeida OP and Flicker L (2003) Preventing dementia: why we should focus on health promotion now. *International Psychogeriatrics*. **15**: 111–19.

2
Epidemiology of dementia

Peter Bowie and Yahya Takriti

Introduction

Dementia has been recognised for thousands of years, being noted in the literature of the Romans and ancient Egyptians and accounts of typical dementia
noted in sources such as *Gulliver's Travels*. Cases were, however, somewhat rare
due to the limited number of individuals reaching an advanced age. As such,
scientific enquiry into the subject was limited. But this is no longer the case. This
chapter will discuss the demographic changes this century, the prevalence and
incidence of dementia and future changes in demography. This chapter will also
discuss the current knowledge of risk factors for dementia and will emphasise
the application of epidemiology and take a global as well as developed world
view. However, first it is necessary to define dementia and its classification.

Definitions of dementia

There have been various attempts to define dementia. For example, Roth[1]
proposed that dementia is 'an acquired global impairment of intellect, memory
and personality'. A more comprehensive definition has been suggested by
McLean:[2] 'An acquired decline in a range of cognitive abilities (memory, learning, orientation and attention) and intellectual skills (abstraction, judgement,
comprehension, language and calculation), accompanied by alterations in personality and behaviour which impair daily functioning, social skills and emotional
control. There is no clouding of consciousness, and other psychiatric disorders
are excluded.' The use of the term 'decline' is helpful because it emphasises the
need for longitudinal assessment and a change from pre-morbid function.
McKhann *et al.*[3] define dementia as 'the decline of memory and other cognitive
functions in comparison with the patient's previous level of function as determined by a history of decline in performance and by abnormalities noted from
clinical examination and neuro-psychological tests'. In addition, they suggest that
diagnosis cannot be made when 'consciousness is impaired by delirium, drowsiness, stupor or coma, or when other clinical abnormalities prevent adequate
evaluation of mental status'. More recently, definitions have been included in
standardised diagnostic criteria, including the American Psychiatric Association's

Diagnostic and Statistical Manual of Mental Disorders (4e) (DSM-IV)[4] and the *International Classification of Diseases (10e) (ICD-10)*.[5] In the *ICD-10* definition, dementia is defined as 'a syndrome due to disease of the brain, usually of a chronic or progressive nature, in which there is disturbance of multiple higher cortical functions, including memory, thinking, orientation, comprehension, calculation, learning capacity, language and judgement. Consciousness is not clouded. Impairments of cognitive function are commonly accompanied, and occasionally preceded, by deterioration in emotional control, social behaviour or motivation.'

Dementia can be classified in a number of different ways. For example, dementia can broadly be classified into reversible and irreversible forms. The irreversible dementias include early and late onset Alzheimer's disease, various forms of vascular dementia including multi-infarct dementia, Pick's disease, Creutzfeldt–Jakob disease, and dementia associated with Huntington's and Parkinson's disease and HIV.[5] These forms of dementia are progressive and usually lead to death. Traditionally, Alzheimer's disease has been thought to account for approximately 50% of all cases of dementia, with multi-infarct dementia and mixed dementia (Alzheimer's disease and multi-infarct dementia combined) each accounting for approximately 20% of all cases; the remaining 10% are due to reversible causes of dementia and less common primary brain degenerative diseases. The variation in the rates for underlying cause is often accounted for by the criteria used for diagnosis, for example the NINDS-AIREN criteria for vascular dementia are more stringent than the *ICD-10* or *DSM-IV* criteria and therefore a lower rate is reported when these criteria are used. It is also worth noting that there is a discrepancy between clinical diagnosis and pathological diagnosis.[6] In the last decade there has been increasing interest in dementia with Lewy bodies, a condition characterised by fluctuating cognitive impairment, prominent hallucinations, parkinsonism and falls. The condition is progressive and has pathological findings similar to Parkinson's disease.[7] It has been suggested that dementia with Lewy bodies is more common than vascular dementia.

A smaller number of patients have 'reversible dementia'. The percentage of dementia patients with a reversible cause has varied from 8%[8] to 40%.[9] Byrne[10] defines reversible dementia as 'the dementia syndrome that is caused by a potentially reversible or treatable condition'.

The potential reversibility of dementia is related to the underlying pathology and to the availability and application of effective treatment. The reversibility will be dependent on the initiating of treatment prior to irreversible damage occurring. Equally, some causes may be arrestable rather than reversible.

The ageing population

Since dementia is primarily a disease of the elderly, a clear understanding of the demographics of ageing can be used to facilitate projections of the epidemiology of dementia and allow for planning of services to meet future needs. The growth of elderly populations poses challenges to services which must adapt provision to provide for the changing age structures of society.

The global population aged 65 and over was estimated to be 420 million in the year 2000, representing an increase of 9.5 million since 1999.[11] In 1990, 26 nations had elderly populations of more than two million and by 2000, 31 countries had reached the two million figure. Projections to the year 2030 indicate that more than 60 nations will have in excess of two million people aged 65 or over.[11] Table 2.1 shows estimates of the percentage of the population aged 65 and over by world region and projections from 2000 to 2030.

Percentages alone do not express a sense of the momentum of population growth. For example, while the projected increase in elderly populations in Sub-Saharan Africa from 2000 to 2015 is only 0.3%, this actually represents an increase of 9.6 million from an elderly population of 19.3 to 28.9 million.

From 1970 to 1996 the percentage of the elderly population of Japan grew from

Table 2.1   Percentage of the population aged 65 and over by world region

Region	Year	65 years +
Europe	2000	15.5
	2015	18.7
	2030	24.3
North America	2000	12.6
	2015	14.9
	2030	20.3
Oceania	2000	10.2
	2015	12.4
	2030	16.3
Asia	2000	6.0
	2015	7.8
	2030	12.0
Latin America/Caribbean	2000	5.5
	2015	7.5
	2030	11.6
Near East/North Africa	2000	4.3
	2015	5.3
	2030	8.1
Sub-Saharan Africa	2000	2.9
	2015	3.2
	2030	3.7

7% to 14%. Similar rapid increases are expected in South Korea, Taiwan, Thailand and China, fuelled by dramatic drops in fertility levels. This speed of change can be contrasted with Europe and North America where comparable increases took place over 100 years.

Increases in life expectancy partly account for the changing demographics of the elderly. This, in conjunction with lowering birth rates, results in a higher proportion of the population being aged 65 and over. Expansion of public health-care and disease eradication programmes greatly increased life expectancy in the second half of the twentieth century, and from 1900 to 1950 people in the developed world were able to add 20 years or more to their life expectancy.[11] Throughout the world there are variations in life expectancy, with people in Japan and Singapore being currently expected to live the longest, around 80 years, whilst many African countries stand at only 45 years.[11] Life expectancy for someone born today in the developed world is, on average, 70.9 years, with the UK standing at 77.7 years and the US at 77.1 years. The average life expectancy for someone born in the developing world is harder to summarise, with estimates ranging from 80.1 years in Singapore (currently the highest) to 37.6 years in Malawi and Zimbabwe.

In general, women outlive men. The UK Census 2001 revealed that the life expectancy of a female born in the UK in 2001 was 80 years, with males expecting to live 75 years.[12] Similar age-related differences were found worldwide.[11] Recent data suggest the gap may be closing in the UK.

In summary, the world's population aged 65 and over is growing by approximately 800 000 people per month.[11] Global ageing is occurring at a pace never seen before, and this rapid increase will be reflected in the epidemiology of age-related diseases such as dementia. One prediction for Alzheimer's disease in the US is that the population affected will quadruple in the next 50 years.[13]

Prevalence and incidence of dementia

Prevalence refers to the number of people with dementia at the given point in time.[14] Prevalence rates vary enormously and some of the reasons for this have been reviewed by Henderson and Kay.[15] As the sample size increases, prevalence estimates become more accurate. Prevalence is also influenced by the sample composition. For example, community samples generally give lower prevalence rates compared with residential homes since the latter tend to cater specifically for patients with dementia. The number of elderly and very elderly in the denominator is also an important factor.

As the number of elderly people in the general population increases, so does the prevalence of dementia, with rates rising from 2.1% between 65–69 years to 17.7% in those aged 80 years or above. Thus, prevalence rates will vary depending on the geographical location of the study. For similar reasons, they will also be influenced by when the study was conducted because the number of elderly in the general population has been gradually increasing over the last 100 years. Diagnostic criteria are also very important in that the more rigid the diagnostic criteria become, the smaller the prevalence of the condition. Finally, the type of prevalence study has a major effect on the prevalence rate. Period prevalence (the number of cases in a given population during a specified period) compared with point prevalence studies (the number of cases in a given population at a specific time) will produce higher prevalence rates since period prevalence is technically a combination of prevalence and incidence.

Incidence is the number of new cases occurring in a given population during a specified time period,[14] and is generally regarded as a more useful indicator than prevalence. This is partly because differences in prevalence rates could be due to either differences in the numbers of new cases or differences in survival rates. Despite this, there have been considerably fewer studies of incidence. Incidence rate is relatively small and in order to yield reliable data, studies either need to be very large or conducted over many years. A review and meta-analysis of studies[16] showed that incidence rates increase with increasing age, but the incidence rate ratio (the rate of change of the incidence) slows down with increasing age, e.g. the incident rate triples from 60 to 65 years, but increases by only a factor of 1.5 from 80 to 85 years. The incidence rate ratio does not fall below 1 so there is no evidence that the rate eventually begins to decline. The incidence rates for five-year age groups are shown in Table 2.2. The reason for the levelling off of the incidence of dementia in the very old is unknown.

Gender does not appear to be a significant factor in the incidence of dementia; women are at higher risk for developing an incidence of Alzheimer's disease whilst men are at higher risk for vascular dementia.[16]

Table 2.2   Annual incidence of dementia from 12 studies[16]

Age group	Annual incidence rate (%)
55–59	0.033
60–64	0.11
65–69	0.33
70–74	0.84
75–79	1.82
80–84	3.36
85–89	5.33
90–94	7.23

Prevalence by age

The exact prevalence of dementia is unknown and is influenced by a number of different factors. Kay and Bergman[17] reported that the prevalence of dementia gradually increases with increasing age: 2.1% are affected between the ages of 65–69 and this rises to 17.7% in those aged 80 or above. Jorm and Jolley[18] suggest, following a meta-analysis of 23 studies, that the prevalence rises exponentially with age, doubling with each successive period of 5.1 years. These findings were confirmed in later studies.[19–21] A summary of the prevalence rates is shown in Table 2.3. There are some inconsistencies concerning prevalence of dementia in extreme old age (aged 90 onwards). Jorm[22] suggested that the risk of developing dementia declines in extreme old age. However, later, Jorm and Jolley[18] found no decrease in extreme old age, suggesting that everybody will develop dementia if they live long enough.

Table 2.3   Age-specific prevalence of dementia averaged from 18 studies[18]

Age group	Prevalence rate (%)
65–69	1.4
70–74	2.8
75–79	5.6
80–84	10.5
85–89	20.8
90–95	38.6

Prevalence by gender

There is invariably a preponderance of females in any demented population, though this largely reflects the greater number of elderly females in the general population. Indeed, the excess of females in 'post-mortem confirmed Alzheimer's disease' is consistent with the age-matched male to female ratio in the general population.[23] Overall, there was no age-specific sex differences in prevalence rates for dementia. However, the prevalence rate of Alzheimer's disease is generally higher amongst females when compared with males of the same age.[24]

Prevalence by geographical area

The reported prevalence and incidence of dementia varies enormously throughout the world. These differences may, in part, be explained by methodological differences, including different diagnostic criteria, screening methods and statistical analyses. However, these differences may also be explained by true differences in the incidence of dementia, the progress of the disease and differential survival rates. Although a great deal of work has been done throughout the world, research conducted in the UK and Ireland, the United States and developing countries including the Far East and Africa will be discussed in more detail in the following sections.

United Kingdom and Ireland

The first major study of the prevalence of dementia in the UK was undertaken by Sheldon[25] in Wolverhampton following World War II. More recent studies have been undertaken in Newcastle,[26] London[27] and Dublin.[28] The prevalence rates obtained vary significantly from 2.3% of 65–70 year-olds to 17.5% of over 80 year-olds. It appears, however, that this variation in prevalence is partly due to differences in the prevalence of different types of dementia, with the onset age for vascular dementia being lower than that of Alzheimer's disease.[29] An overall rate of 5% is suggested in the population over 65 years of age.[30]

United States

Similar rates to those obtained in the UK have been seen in North America,[31] with approximately 5% of those aged over 65 suffering from dementia.

In the US, an interesting area of research is ethnic differences. The majority of studies in the US have, however, focused on predominantly white populations. An exception to this is a study by Perkins et al.[32] who screened white, Hispanic and black retired men in Houston. They found a difference in the prevalence of dementia relating to ethnic group. Hispanic and black men were found to be at highest risk, with prevalence of 4.75% and 4.80% respectively, whilst white men had a prevalence of 2.42%. However, it should be noted that a higher incidence of stroke, hypertension and diabetes are found in African-Americans and this could partly account for the higher prevalence of dementia, especially given that the Perkins et al. study[32] found 55% of their participants being diagnosed with vascular dementia, with only 20% having Alzheimer's disease. More detailed work is required, therefore, to fully understand the link between ethnicity and geographical area with respect to dementia.

Developing countries: the Far East

An interesting pattern has been obtained in the Far East. In the past, Chinese culture has associated the appearance of dementia with retribution for past sins, the imbalance of yin and yang, and a consequence of astrological activity.[33] Such beliefs may result in dementia being seen not as an illness, and the help of Chinese healers rather than westernised medical help being sought. Rapid urbanisation is, however, being shown to be resulting in changing family structure in the Far East, such as smaller family sizes in China, and the beliefs regarding dementia have also been shown to be becoming more 'westernised'.[33]

Many early studies on dementia in the Far East yielded low prevalence rates.[34] More recent studies, however, adopting a rigorous methodology, indicated a prevalence rate of around 5%.[35,36] The majority of the work has focused on urban populations with the rural population of China, for example, totalling one billion, yet to be surveyed. The inclusion of this population could change the estimates of prevalence.

Japan, a country with one of the highest life expectancies, had one million dementia sufferers in 1990, and the number of sufferers was estimated to double by 2010.[37] The incidence of vascular dementia in Japan[38] was greater than the incidence of Alzheimer's disease, with double the rate for men and similar rates for women. More recently, Yamada et al.[39] have found that this picture has reversed and Alzheimer's disease is twice as prevalent as vascular dementia. In addition they also found a significant number of cases of dementia with Lewy bodies, but these did not match the rates for vascular dementia.

Developing countries: Africa

The majority of the work on dementia in Africa has been conducted in Nigeria. Research has included community surveys, hospital admission studies and autopsy studies. Three separate community surveys, with approximately 23 000 participants have found no cases of dementia.[40–42] It has been suggested that the nil rate may be due to a number of different factors, particularly the lower life expectancy, also African families being tolerant of disturbed behaviour, a reluctance to seek psychiatrists' help, a preference for the use of African medicine and a fear of stigmatisation. Recently, American psychiatrists conducted a study that found a prevalence rate of 2.29% for dementia, and 1.41% for Alzheimer's alone.[43] Interestingly, however, this study was extended to include a comparison group of Nigerians living in the United States. Significantly higher prevalence rates for dementia and Alzheimer's disease were obtained for the US Nigerian population of 8.24% and 6.24% respectively.[44] This finding suggests the involvement of environmental factors in the detection and possibly aetiology of dementia.

Temporal changes in the prevalence of dementia

Two major studies have investigated the prevalence of dementia over time. The Lundby study in Sweden followed prevalence of dementia from 1947 to 1972, and showed no change in prevalence of either multi-infarct or what was described as 'senile dementia'.[45] Similarly, no change in prevalence was obtained in Rochester, US from 1975 to 1980.[46] However, Kokmen et al.[47] found an increase in the cases of dementia in Rochester between 1960 and 1984.

Suh and Shah[48] conducted a meta-analysis of all publications on the epidemiology of dementia from 1966 to 1999. Overall they concluded that the prevalence of dementia had increased and it appeared that when dementia was separated into Alzheimer's disease and vascular dementia for the purposes of analysis, temporal changes could be seen. The prevalence of the two types was found to vary throughout the world. Although these differences may be partly due to methodological differences, they may, however, reflect true differences in the incidence, differential survival and mortality after the onset of dementia. A difference in the prevalence of dementia in Korea, China and Japan was observed, with vascular dementia being more common in the 1980s whilst Alzheimer's disease was more common in the 1990s.

Risk factors for dementia

As we have already discussed, the prevalence of dementia and especially Alzheimer's disease increases exponentially with increasing age, thus age is by far the biggest risk factor for dementia. Relatively few risk factors have been conclusively established, although many have been considered. Most of the evidence on risk factors has been based on case–control studies, but large longitudinal cohort studies have now been published which avoid some of the methodological problems associated with case–control studies.

Family history of Alzheimer's disease and other dementias has been associated with a risk for Alzheimer's disease in most studies, but not all. A number of genes have been identified as being associated with Alzheimer's disease: mutations of genes on chromosomes 1, 14 and 21 are linked with early-onset familial Alzheimer's disease, but together these genes account for fewer than 2% of all cases. The vast majority of cases are late-onset and so far the only confirmed genetic marker associated with late-onset risk is the ε4 allele of apolipoprotein E (APOE), a protein encoded on chromosome 19.[49] There are three allelic variants of APOE ε: these are ε2, ε3, and ε4. ε3 is the most frequent allele found in the general population with frequency estimates ranging from 63–85%; ε2 is comparatively rare (3–13%) and ε4 frequencies range from 7–29%. People who are ε4 homozygotes (possess two ε4 alleles) are at particular risk of developing Alzheimer's disease, with 50–90% of such individuals eventually developing the disease. Those with one ε4 allele also carry an increased risk, with 29% eventually developing the disease. Those individuals without the ε4 allele have a lifetime risk of about 9%.[50] Homozygosity for APOE ε4 has also been linked to a faster rate of cognitive decline, suggesting that the protein has a mechanistic role in disease progression and is not simply related to disease onset.[51]

There is substantial evidence that a history of head injury increases the risk of Alzheimer's disease, though some studies have not found an association.[52,53] It has been well established that head injury is associated with a massive increase in amyloid in the brain, and it is the brain's ability to deal with this increased amyloid burden that is the likely mechanism for any increased risk.

Other factors associated with increased risk of Alzheimer's disease are less well established. Family history of brain disease and parental age has both been studied; both reflect possible exposure to genetic factors. Family histories of Parkinson's disease and Down's syndrome have been studied with inconsistent results.[54,55] Likewise, maternal age at birth has not consistently been associated with an increased risk of dementia. Other medical conditions such as allergic conditions, hypothyroidism and viral infection do not have a consistent association with Alzheimer's disease.[56]

Environmental and lifestyle factors have also been studied. Aluminium has been researched for many years, but there is still not conclusive evidence that it has a causal role in Alzheimer's disease.[57] Smoking has been widely studied: earlier case–control studies suggested that smoking may reduce the risk of Alzheimer's disease but more recent longitudinal cohort studies have shown no effect or an increased risk.[58] A study looking at the combined effect of smoking, drinking and exercise suggested that these factors were not associated with risk of Alzheimer's disease.[59] Results from a Canadian cohort study involving over 6000 subjects suggested that regular physical activity and use of wine, coffee and NSAIDs were associated with a reduced risk of Alzheimer's disease;[60] the authors suggested that these factors required further investigation.

Vascular risk factors such as hypertension, hypercholesterolaemia and atherosclerosis have been shown to increase the risk of Alzheimer's disease and dementia generally.[61]

Other factors have been associated with a reduced risk of developing Alzheimer's disease. The most consistent evidence is regarding higher educational attainment and length of education, which are associated with a lower risk.[62] The use of various medications and vitamins has been explored. Large longitudinal studies have shown a significantly reduced risk for Alzheimer's disease with anti-inflammatory drugs, statins, hormone replacement therapy (HRT) and vitamins C and E. A prospective cohort study of nearly 7000 subjects followed up for seven years[63] found that short-term use of NSAIDs was associated with a relative risk of Alzheimer's disease of 0.95, whilst long-term use was associated with a relative risk of 0.2. Use of NSAIDs did not reduce the risk of vascular dementia. In a nested case–control study,[64] the authors found that the adjusted relative risk (odds ratio) of developing dementia was 0.29 for those prescribed statins. This finding was independent of the presence or absence of untreated hyperlipidaemia. In a review of HRT, Fillit[65] concluded that most evidence indicates that HRT mitigates the degeneration that leads to Alzheimer's disease. At present there is no evidence to suggest that HRT is of benefit once Alzheimer's disease is clinically apparent. Two large longitudinal cohort studies recently published in the *Journal of the American Medical Association* suggested that antioxidant use (vitamins C and E) was associated with a reduced risk of Alzheimer's disease. Engelhart *et al.*[66] followed up over 5000 participants for six years and found, after adjusting for confounders, a significantly reduced risk in those using vitamin C and vitamin E: this finding was independent of APOE ε status. The other study[67] followed a cohort of 815 participants for nearly four years and found that increased vitamin E intake was associated with a lower risk of Alzheimer's disease; however, this finding was only observed in those people who were APOE ε4 negative.

Lastly there is the question of depression, which is associated with cognitive impairment in older people.[68] Case–control studies have suggested an association between a history of depression and risk of Alzheimer's disease.[69] However longitudinal studies have been inconsistent.[70,71]

Discussion

A major problem in epidemiological studies of dementia is defining a case. This is especially true for mild cases of dementia, particularly when combined with poor education or lower IQ.[72] In addition, there are difficulties when using informants,[73] which may be particularly true in developing countries. Informants may have a tendency to offer responses perceived to be acceptable to the interviewer, may expect questions to be addressed to the head of the family/tribe, and personal questions may be avoided. In developing countries, reporting of age has been shown to be inaccurate, with under-reporting by three years being observed in elderly Indian patients[74] while Chinese informants tend to add an extra year.[75]

Some techniques of case identification are less reliable than others. For example, hospital admission is not a reliable index of dementia cases as the majority of patients are likely to be nursed at home, particularly in developing countries. Geographical comparison based on hospital admission is a reflection of service provision rather than prevalence of dementia.[76]

Despite such methodological concerns, the study of the epidemiology of dementia is crucial. As the age distribution of the world population shifts, dementia is emerging as a major health problem. The assessment of epidemiology of the disease provides crucial input for public health professionals in determining and allocating healthcare resources. The increasing burden of care for families has to be taken on by governmental response. Issues to be addressed by governments include the extent of domiciliary, day and residential care that should be available in order to provide the appropriate level of support for both sufferers and their families. Due to the increasing life expectancy, the number of people suffering from dementia will rise steeply over the next decades. Additional importance must be given to planning for the care of the elderly, and to account for the likely dramatic increase of dementia sufferers in the future. In addition, strategies to reduce risk must be sought, evaluated and implemented. Dementia can be seen as a problem today and a likely epidemic tomorrow.

Key points

- The work reviewed in this chapter provides an overview of the prevalence and incidence of dementia across the world, and considers possible risk factors associated with disease onset.
- Epidemiology has enormous potential for identifying modifiable risk factors and ways to prevent disease.
- Further advances in the understanding of dementia are required, and epidemiological studies have been of use in providing such insights.
- Further intensive studies into areas where rates appear very high or low may prove fruitful in furthering research into the aetiology of dementia.

References

1   Roth M (1955) The natural history of mental disorder in old age. *Journal of Mental Science.* **101**: 281–301.
2   McLean S (1987) Assessing dementia. Part 1: Difficulties, definitions and differential diagnosis. *Australian and New Zealand Journal of Psychiatry.* **21**: 142–74.
3   McKhann G, Drachman D, Folstein M *et al.* (1984) Clinical diagnosis of Alzheimer's disease: report of the NINCDS-ADRDA Work Group under the

auspices of the Department of Health and Human Services Task Force on Alzheimer's Disease. *Neurology.* **34**: 939–44.

4 American Psychiatric Association (1994) *Diagnostic and Statistical Manual of Mental Disorders* (4e). APA, Washington, DC.

5 World Health Organization (1992) *The ICD-10 Classification of Mental and Behavioural Disorders: clinical descriptions and diagnostic guidelines.* WHO, Geneva.

6 Knopman DS, DeKosky ST, Cummings JL *et al.* (2001) Practice parameter: diagnosis of dementia (an evidence-based review). Report of the Quality Standards Subcommittee of the American Academy of Neurology. *Neurology.* **56**: 1143–53.

7 McKeith IG, Galasko D, Kosaka K *et al.* (1996) Consensus guidelines for the clinical and pathologic diagnosis of dementia with Lewy bodies (DLB): report of the consortium on DLB international workshop. *Neurology.* **47**: 1113–24.

8 Pearce J and Miller E (1973) *Clinical Aspects of Dementia.* Bailliere Tindall, London.

9 Hutton JT (1981) Senility reconsidered. *Journal of the American Medical Association.* **245**: 1025–6.

10 Byrne EJ (1987) Diffuse Lewy body disease: disease spectrum disorder or variety of Alzheimer's disease? *International Journal of Geriatric Psychiatry.* **7**: 229–34.

11 Kinsella K and Velkoff V (2001) *An Ageing World: 2001.* International population reports: US Department of Health and Human Sciences, National Institute of Health. United States Census Bureau, Washington, DC.

12 Office for National Statistics (2001) *Social Trends.* HMSO, London.

13 Brookmeyer R, Gray S and Kawas C (1998) Projections of Alzheimer's disease in the United States and the public health impact of delaying disease onset. *American Journal of Public Health.* **88**: 1337–42.

14 Barker DJP and Rose G (1990) *Epidemiology in Medical Practice* (4e). Churchill Livingstone, London.

15 Henderson AS and Kay DWK (1984) The epidemiology of mental disorders in the aged. In: DWK Kay and GD Burrows (eds) *Handbook of Studies on Psychiatry and Old Age.* Elsevier, Amsterdam.

16 Gao S, Hendrie HC, Hall KS *et al.* (1998) The relationships between age, sex, and the incidence of dementia and Alzheimer disease: a meta-analysis. *Archives of General Psychiatry.* **55**: 809–15.

17 Kay DWK and Bergman K (1980) Epidemiology of mental disorders among the aged in the community. In: JE Birren and RB Sloane (eds) *Handbook of Mental Health and Ageing.* Prentice-Hall, Englewood Cliffs, NJ.

18 Jorm AF and Jolley D (1998) The incidence of dementia: a meta-analysis. *Neurology.* **51**(3): 728–33.

19 Rocca WA, Hofman A, Brayne C *et al.* (1991) Frequency and distribution of Alzheimer's disease in Europe: a collaborative study of 1980–1990 prevalence findings. The EURODEM Prevalence Research Group. *Annals of Neurology.* **30**: 381–90.

20 Copeland JRM, Davidson IA, Dewey ME *et al.* (1992) Alzheimer's disease,

other dementias, depression and pseudo-dementia: prevalence, incidence and three year outcome in Liverpool. *British Journal of Psychiatry.* **161**: 230–39.

21 von Strauss E, Viitanen M, De Ronchi D *et al.* (1999) Aging and the occurrence of dementia: findings from a population-based cohort with a large sample of nonagenarians. *Archives of Neurology.* **56**: 587–92.

22 Jorm AF (1991) Cross-national comparisons of the occurrence of Alzheimer's and vascular dementias. *European Archives of Psychiatry and Clinical Neuroscience.* **240**: 218–22.

23 Heston LL, Mastri AR, Anderson VW *et al.* (1981) Dementia of the Alzheimer type. Clinical genetics, natural history and associated conditions. *Archives of General Psychiatry.* **38**: 1085–90.

24 Jorm AF, Korten AE and Henderson AS (1987) The prevalence of dementia: a quantitative integration of the literature. *Acta Psychiatrica Scandinavica.* **76**: 465–79.

25 Sheldon JH (1948) *The Social Medicine of Old Age.* Oxford University Press, London.

26 Newens AJ, Forster DP, Kay DW *et al.* (1993) Clinically diagnosed presenile dementia of the Alzheimer type in the Northern health region: ascertainment, prevalence, incidence and survival. *Psychological Medicine.* **23**: 631–44.

27 Livingstone G, Hawkins A and Graham N (1990) The Gospel Oak study: prevalence rates of dementia and depression and activity limitation among elderly residents in inner London. *Psychological Medicine.* **20**: 137–46.

28 Lawler BA, Radic A and Bruce I (1994) Prevalence of mental illness in an elderly community dwelling population using AGECAT. *Irish Journal of Psychological Medicine.* **11**: 157–9.

29 Brayne C and Calloway P (1989) An epidemiological study of dementia in a rural population of elderly women. *British Journal of Psychiatry.* **155**: 214–19.

30 Ineichen B (1998) The geography of dementia: an approach through epidemiology. *Health and Place.* **4**(4): 383–94.

31 Henderson AS (1994) *Dementia.* World Health Organization, Geneva.

32 Perkins P, Annegars JF, Doody RS *et al.* (1997) Incidence and prevalence of dementia in a multi-ethnic cohort of municipal retirees. *Neurology.* **49**(1): 44–50.

33 Elliott KS, Di Minno M and Lam D (1996) Working with Chinese families in the context of dementia. In: G Yeo and D Gallagher-Thompson (eds) *Ethnicity and the Dementias,* pp. 89–108. Taylor and Francis, Washington, DC.

34 Kua EH (1991) The prevalence of dementia in elderly Chinese. *Acta Psychiatrica Scandinavica.* **83**: 350–2.

35 Chiu HFK, Pang AHT, Lam LCW *et al.* (1996) Letter from Hong Kong. *International Journal of Geriatric Psychiatry.* **11**: 711–13.

36 Yang C-H, Hwang J-P and Tsai S-J (1996) Types and phenomenologic subtypes of dementia in Taiwan: a psychiatric inpatient study. *International Journal of Geriatric Psychiatry.* **11**: 705–9.

37 Ineichen B (1996) Senile dementia in Japan: prevalence and response. *Society for Scientific Medicine.* **42**(2): 169–72.

38 Yoshitake T, Kiyohara Y, Kato I *et al.* (1995) Incidence and risk factors of vascular dementia and Alzheimer's disease in a defined elderly Japanese population: the Hisayama Study. *Neurology.* **45**: 1161–8.

39 Yamada T, Hattori H, Miura A *et al.* (2001) Prevalence of Alzheimer's disease, vascular dementia and dementia with Lewy bodies in a Japanese population. *Psychiatry and Clinical Neurosciences.* **55**: 21–5.

40 Osuntokun BO, Adeuja AOG, Schoenberg BS *et al.* (1987) Neurological disorders in Nigerian Africans: a community based study. *Acta Neurologica Scandinavica.* **75**: 13.

41 Longe AC and Osuntokun BO (1989) Prevalence of neurological disorders in Udo, a rural community in Southern Nigeria. *Tropical Geography Medicine.* **41**: 36–40.

42 Ogunniyi AO, Osuntokun BO, Lekwauwa UB *et al.* (1992) Rarity of dementia (by DSM-III-R) in an urban community in Nigeria. *East African Medical Journal.* **69**(2): 64–8.

43 Hendrie HC, Osuntokun BO, Hall KS *et al.* (1995) Prevalence of Alzheimer's disease and dementia in two communities: Nigerian Africans and African-Americans. *American Journal of Psychiatry.* **152**(10): 1485–92.

44 Ogunniyi A, Baiyewu O, Gureje O *et al.* (2000) Epidemiology of dementia in Nigeria: results from the Indianapolis–Ibadan study. *European Journal of Neurology.* **7**: 485–90.

45 Roorsman B, Hagnell O and Lanke J (1986) Prevalence and incidence of senile and multi-infarct dementia in the Lundby study: a comparison between the time periods 1947–1957 and 1957–1972. *Neuropsychobiology.* **15**: 122–9.

46 Beard CM, Kokmen E, Offord K *et al.* (1991) Is the prevalence of dementia changing? *Neurology.* **41**: 1911–14.

47 Kokmen E, Beard CM, O'Brien PC *et al.* (1993) Is the incidence of dementing illness changing? A 25-year time trend study in Rochester, Minnesota (1960–1984). *Neurology.* **43**: 1887–92.

48 Suh G-H and Shah A (2001) A review of the epidemiological transition in dementia: cross-national comparisons of the indices related to Alzheimer's disease and vascular dementia. *Acta Psychiatrica Scandinavica.* **104**(1): 4–11.

49 Farrer LA, Cupples LA, Haines JL *et al.* (1997) Effects of age, sex, and ethnicity on the association between apolipoprotein E genotype and Alzheimer disease. A meta-analysis. APOE and Alzheimer Disease Meta-Analysis Consortium. *Journal of the American Medical Association.* **278**: 1349–56.

50 Seshadri S, Drachman DA and Lippa CF (1995) Apolipoprotein E epsilon 4 allele and the lifetime risk of Alzheimer's disease. What physicians know, and what they should know. *Archives of Neurology.* **52**: 1074–9.

51 Craft S, Teri L, Edland SD *et al.* (1998) Accelerated decline in apolipoprotein E epsilon 4 homozygotes with Alzheimer's disease. *Neurology.* **51**: 149–53.

52 Mortimer JA, van Duijn CM, Chandra V *et al.* (1991) Head trauma as a risk factor for Alzheimer's disease: a collaborative re-analysis of case–control studies. EURODEM Risk Factors Research Group. *International Journal of Epidemiology.* **20** (Suppl 2): 28–35.

53 Launer LJ, Andersen K, Dewey ME *et al.* (1999) Rates and risk factors for dementia and Alzheimer's disease: results from EURODEM pooled analyses. *Neurology.* **52**(1): 78–84.

54 van Duijn CM, Clayton D, Chandra V *et al.* (1991) Familial aggregation of Alzheimer's disease and related disorders: a collaborative re-analysis of case–

control studies. EURODEM Risk Factors Research Group. *International Journal of Epidemiology*. **20** (Suppl 2): 13–20.

55 Fratiglioni L, Ahlbom A, Viitanen M *et al.* (1993) Risk factors for late-onset Alzheimer's disease: a population-based, case–control study. *Annals of Neurology*. **33**: 258–66.

56 Graves AB, White E, Koepsell TD *et al.* (1990) A case–control study of Alzheimer's disease. *Annals of Neurology*. **28**: 766–74.

57 Doll R (1993) Review: Alzheimer's disease and environmental aluminium. *Age and Ageing*. **22**: 138–53.

58 Wang HX, Fratiglioni L, Frisoni GB *et al.* (1999) Smoking and the occurrence of Alzheimer's disease: cross-sectional and longitudinal data in a population-based study. *American Journal of Epidemiology*. **149**: 640–4.

59 Broe GA, Creasey H, Jorm AF *et al.* (1998) Health habits and risk of cognitive impairment and dementia in old age: a prospective study on the effects of exercise, smoking and alcohol consumption. *Australian and New Zealand Journal of Public Health*. **22**: 621–3.

60 Lindsay J, Laurin D, Verreault R *et al.* (2002) Risk factors for Alzheimer's disease: a prospective analysis from the Canadian Study of Health and Aging. *American Journal of Epidemiology*. **156**: 445–53.

61 Hofman A, Ott A, Breteler MM *et al.* (1997) Atherosclerosis, apolipoprotein E, and prevalence of dementia and Alzheimer's disease in the Rotterdam Study. *Lancet*. **349**: 151–4.

62 Katzman R (1993) Education and the prevalence of dementia and Alzheimer's disease. *Neurology*. **43**: 13–20.

63 in t'Veld BA, Ruitenberg A, Hofman A *et al.* (2001) Non-steroidal anti-inflammatory drugs and the risk of Alzheimer's disease. *New England Journal of Medicine*. **345**: 1515–21.

64 Jick H, Zornberg GL, Jick SS *et al.* (2000) Statins and the risk of dementia. *Lancet*. **356**: 1627–31.

65 Fillit HM (2002) The role of hormone replacement therapy in the prevention of Alzheimer disease. *Archives of Internal Medicine*. **162**: 1934–42.

66 Engelhart MJ, Geerlings MI, Ruitenberg A *et al.* (2002) Dietary intake of antioxidants and risk of Alzheimer disease. *Journal of the American Medical Association*. **287**: 3223–9.

67 Morris MC, Evans DA, Bienias JL *et al.* (2002) Dietary intake of antioxidant nutrients and the risk of incident Alzheimer disease in a biracial community study. *Journal of the American Medical Association*. **287**: 3230–7.

68 Burt DB, Zembar MJ and Niederehe G (1995) Depression and memory impairment: a meta-analysis of the association, its pattern, and specificity. *Psychological Bulletin*. **117**: 285–305.

69 Jorm AF, van Duijn CM, Chandra V *et al.* (1991) Psychiatric history and related exposures as risk factors for Alzheimer's disease: a collaborative re-analysis of case–control studies. EURODEM Risk Factors Research Group. *International Journal of Epidemiology*. **20** (Suppl 2): 43–7.

70 Chen P, Ganguli M, Mulsant BH *et al.* (1999) The temporal relationship between depressive symptoms and dementia: a community-based prospective study. *Archives of General Psychiatry*. **56**: 261–6.

71 Schmand B, Jonker C, Geerlings MI *et al.* (1997) Subjective memory complaints in the elderly: depressive symptoms and future dementia. *British Journal of Psychiatry.* **171**: 373–6.

72 Prencipe M, Casini AR and Ferretti C (1996) Prevalence of dementia in an elderly rural population: effects of age, sex and education. *Journal of Neurology, Neurosurgery and Psychiatry.* **60**: 628–33.

73 Pollitt PA (1996) Dementia in old age: an anthropological perspective. *Psychological Medicine.* **26**: 1061–74.

74 Srinivasan TN, Suresh TR and Rajkumar S (1993) Age estimation in the elderly: relevance to geriatric research in developing countries. *Indian Journal of Psychiatry.* **35**(1): 58–9.

75 Kua EH, Ko SM, Fones SLC *et al.* (1996) Comorbidity of depression in the elderly: an epidemiological study in a Chinese community. *International Journal of Geriatric Psychiatry.* **11**: 699–704.

76 Bamforth G and Ineichen B (1996) How to add insult to carers' injuries. *Journal of Dementia Care.* **4**(2): 14–15.

3
Diagnosis and classification

Anna V Richman and Ken CM Wilson

Introduction

Dementia has been defined as 'an acquired global impairment of intellect, memory and personality...'.[1] It is usually progressive and irreversible and can be due to a number of different causes. It generally develops gradually. An intercurrent illness or a change in social circumstances may herald its presentation. Dementia of whatever type is usually more common with increasing age. The general criteria for the diagnosis of dementia are:[2]

- a decline in memory, most evident in the learning of new information
- a decline in other cognitive abilities, characterised by deterioration in judgement and thinking, and in the general processing of information
- a decline in emotional control or motivation, or a change in social behaviour
- the awareness of the environment is preserved during a period of time sufficiently long to allow the demonstration of the above symptoms
- for a confident clinical diagnosis the symptoms should have been present for at least six months.

Causes of dementia

Once a provisional diagnosis of dementia has been made, the clinician needs to clarify the type of dementia from which the person is suffering. The history of how the impairment has developed, along with appropriate tests and examinations, may help to determine the cause. Dementia was classified traditionally as pre-senile or senile, based on age of onset (before or after 65 years of age respectively). The age of onset may be helpful in deciding on the aetiology, but many of the causes of dementia are found in both age groups, making this traditional approach to classification relatively redundant. Alzheimer's disease is the most common cause of dementia. Other common causes include vascular dementia and Lewy body dementia. Mixed Alzheimer's disease and vascular dementia is not uncommon. These dementias are discussed in more detail later in the chapter. A brief description will now be provided about some of the less common types of dementia.

Frontotemporal dementia

The features of this dementia are an early loss of insight, personality change, hyperorality, non-fluent aphasia and well-preserved spatial orientation. Neurological signs are often absent early in the disease, or are limited to the presence of primitive reflexes. There is an equal incidence in men and women and a high familial incidence. Onset occurs most commonly between the ages of 45 and 65 years and the mean duration of illness is eight years.

Dementia in Pick's disease

This is another progressive dementia commencing in middle age. The general criteria for dementia[2] must be met as well as:

- slow onset with steady deterioration

- predominance of frontal lobe involvement, evidenced by at least two of: emotional blunting, coarsening of social behaviour, disinhibition, apathy or restlessness, aphasia

- early on, memory and parietal lobe functions are relatively preserved.

It may be viewed as a form of frontotemporal dementia with specific pathological features at post-mortem.

Dementia in Creutzfeldt–Jakob disease

The onset is usually in middle or later life. Death occurs within one to two years. The general criteria for dementia must be met[2] along with:

- a very rapid progression, with disintegration of virtually all higher cerebral functions

- at least one of the following: pyramidal or extrapyramidal or cerebellar symptoms, aphasia, visual impairment.

Dementia in Huntington's disease

Huntington's disease is inherited in an autosomal dominant pattern. It may present with cognitive problems or a movement disorder. Symptoms typically emerge during the third and fourth decades and progression is slow. There are involuntary choreiform movements, as well as slowness of thinking or movement and personality alteration. Apathy or depression may also be present. There must be a family history of the disease.

Dementia in Parkinson's disease

A dementia may develop in the course of established Parkinson's disease. There are no particular distinguishing features for this type of dementia. However, it is important that none of the cognitive impairment is attributable to any medication that the patient may be using.

Dementia in human immunodeficiency virus (HIV) disease

Patients with a diagnosis of HIV infection may develop a dementia in the course of the disease. This may present with a variety of motor and behavioural changes, which are progressive. HIV dementia is very rare in those with asymptomatic HIV infection, affecting less than 1%. In those with symptomatic HIV disease, the prevalence rises to 10–20%.[3]

Alcoholic dementia

Alcohol is known to be neurotoxic, but the existence of 'alcoholic dementia' as a distinct entity is doubtful. Many patients diagnosed with alcoholic dementia actually have Korsakoff's syndrome (an amnesic syndrome, not a dementia). Few studies have looked at people diagnosed with this dementia. One study has estimated that among alcoholics attending an outpatient facility, over 50% of patients aged over 45 years, with a long history of alcohol abuse, will be found to have some degree of cognitive impairment.[4] Most will have minor impairments of memory or concentration etc., but a few will have a dementia. However, the dementia could be a vascular or Alzheimer type dementia. Perhaps the term 'cognitive impairment in association with alcohol' would be more appropriate.

Other causes of dementia

It is important not to forget about other causes of dementia. Some of these are potentially reversible with treatment, but most show a partial response to treatment. These include:

- infections, e.g. neurosyphilis
- vitamin deficiencies, e.g. B_{12}, folate

- endocrine and metabolic disorders, e.g. hypothyroidism
- drugs
- neoplasms
- normal pressure hydrocephalus
- subdural haematomas.

Causes of dementia – a summary

- *Neurodegenerative*: Alzheimer's; frontotemporal; lewy body.
- *Vascular*: infarction; haemorrhage; vasculitis; Binswanger's disease.
- *Endocrine*: thyroid disease; diabetes; Cushing's disease; Addison's disease; parathyroid disease.
- *Vitamin deficiencies*: B_{12}; thiamine; nicotinic acid.
- *Systemic diseases*: anaemia; respiratory disease; renal disease; hepatic disease.
- *Neurological disorders*: head injury; neoplasms, normal pressure hydrocephalus; Parkinson's disease; Huntington's disease.
- *Infection*: syphilis; HIV.

Subcortical dementia

Over the last 30 years there has been an emerging view that dementia can also be separated into cortical and subcortical types. The differentiating features of subcortical dementia are said to be a profound slowing of cognition, memory disturbances, frontal executive dysfunction, and changes in personality and affect in the absence of aphasias, apraxias and agnosias.[5] Subcortical dementias include those associated with Huntington's disease, Parkinson's disease and HIV. Alzheimer's dementia is the most common cortical dementia. It is well recognised, however, that cortical abnormalities are often found in subcortical diseases and vice versa.

The importance of an accurate diagnosis

Both the progression of the illness and the treatment will vary according to the cause of the dementia. An accurate diagnosis has become particularly important over the last few years with the introduction of acetylcholinesterase inhibitors for use in Alzheimer's disease. It is also an important issue in the treatment of Lewy body dementia where extreme sensitivity to the side-effects of neuroleptic medication is common. Consequently, the cause of the dementia needs to be clarified so that appropriate medication can be used and the course and prognosis better understood. A thorough history and examination of the patient, including relevant investigations (blood tests, brain scans, etc.), will help to determine the cause, and also help to differentiate it from other common conditions such as depression or delirium, which may present in a similar fashion.

Diagnostic criteria

Criteria for the diagnosis of dementia vary between different classification systems. The two main classification systems in use are the American Psychiatric Association's *Diagnostic and Statistical Manual of Mental Disorders* (4e) (*DSM-IV*)[6] and the *International Classification of Diseases* (10e) (*ICD-10*).[2] The general criteria for dementia according to *ICD-10* are summarised as:

- A syndrome due to disease of the brain, usually of a chronic (at least six months) or progressive nature.

- There is a disturbance of memory and other higher cortical functions, including thinking, orientation, comprehension, calculation, learning capacity, language and judgement.

- Consciousness is not clouded.

- The impairments of cognitive function are commonly accompanied by deterioration in emotional control, social behaviour or motivation.

Further criteria may then be applied, specific to each type of dementia.

Alzheimer's dementia

This is the most common cause of dementia in old age and also occurs in those under 65 years of age. It was first described in 1907 by Alois Alzheimer.[7] He described the case of a woman who died aged 51 years with all the symptoms of dementia. This initially led to Alzheimer's disease being thought of as a disease of younger people. Subsequent work has shown that Alzheimer's disease does occur in both older and younger people.[8]

Clinical features

The disease may go unnoticed at first, and is often mistaken for memory changes associated with normal ageing. Intellectual deterioration is slow to develop, but insight is often lost at an early stage. The disease progresses gradually (see Case Study 3.1). The clinical features may be considered in three stages, the patient presenting at any stage.

Case Study 3.1

A 72-year-old lady was seen at home by an old age psychiatrist. The lady herself denied any problems but did admit that her memory was not as good as it used to be. She put this down to old age. Her daughter said that she first noticed her mother's memory problems two years ago and since that time she felt that the problems had got worse. Initially she had difficulty remembering names, telephone numbers, etc., but more recently her mother had got lost on two occasions when she was out doing her shopping. The family had also taken over the preparation of meals after the lady had twice put food in the oven to cook and then forgotten about it, resulting in a smoke-filled kitchen. She had stopped doing the daily crossword and also seemed to have problems dealing with bills and cash. She did not appear to be depressed and was a non-smoker. She had never been in hospital in her life and was not on any medication. There was no family history of any mental health problems. Recent routine blood tests were all normal and a CT scan of her brain showed no evidence of any vascular problems. On examination she scored poorly on tests of her memory, recall and orientation. A diagnosis of Alzheimer's disease was made and she was referred on to the local memory clinic for further assessment and treatment.

Early stage

This generally lasts from two to three years. The clinical features include:

- memory impairment
- difficulties performing everyday tasks
- impaired concentration
- spatial disorientation
- disturbances of mood – depression, euphoria or lability of mood
- fatigue, anxiety and lack of spontaneity.

Some patients maintain good social competence despite severe cognitive impairment.

Intermediate stage

The above features persist and may deteriorate further. Other features may include:

- apraxia and agnosia
- deterioration in reading and writing ability

- disorientation in time and place (may lead to night-time waking and wandering)

- speech problems, e.g. nominal dysphasia

- emotional lability and catastrophic reactions (extreme distress and anxiety when unable to complete a task)

- extrapyramidal disorders, e.g. increased muscle tone and altered gait

- delusions and/or hallucinations.

Late stage

The features of this stage can include:

- double incontinence

- lack of communication

- emaciation

- limb contractures

- grand mal seizures

- primitive reflexes.

The patient often becomes bedridden and death frequently results from a subsequent infection, e.g. a chest infection. Death usually occurs within two to eight years from the onset of the disease. *ICD-10* requires that the general criteria for dementia are met, and that there is no evidence from the history, physical examination or further investigations, e.g. a computed tomography (CT) brain scan, of cerebrovascular disease or any other possible cause of dementia.

There is a large variation in the degree and rate of cognitive decline in patients with Alzheimer's dementia. However, defining the anticipated course of the disease in detail can help patients and their families manage the present and plan for the future. Change can be measured by the rate of decline on cognitive testing and by using staging instruments. Two widely used staging schemes are the Washington University Clinical Dementia Rating (CDR)[9] and the Global Deterioration Scale (GDS).[10]

The GDS divides Alzheimer's disease into seven distinguishable stages. Criteria for many of the stages combine a history (memory problems, self-care, language, gait, etc.) with a mental state examination. The history is mainly obtained from the care-giver. Neither of these scales is sensitive as a measure of short-term change, as movement between stages may take several years. They are used mainly for research or for following patients longitudinally over long time periods.

Risk factors for Alzheimer's disease

Dementia is a common cause of disability and dependency in society today. Over the last two decades there has been much interest and research into the risk factors for Alzheimer's dementia. This is an important area because of the potential implications for the prevention of the disease by modifying the risk factors.

Genes as risk factors

In cases of early-onset Alzheimer's disease (starting before 65 years of age), an association has been found with mutations associated with a number of genes, including those found on chromosomes 21, 14 and 1. The link with chromosome 21 is interesting, given that patients with Down's syndrome (trisomy 21) have a much higher incidence of Alzheimer's disease than the general population. However, these mutations account for only 30–50% of all autosomal dominant early-onset cases.[11] A clear autosomal dominant pattern of inheritance is rare in cases starting after 65 years of age. Many genes have been proposed as having importance as risk factors for late-onset cases, but studies of these genes have often not been replicated. There does, however, seem to be an increased risk associated with the possession of one or more copies of the APOE ε4 allele (found on chromosome 19) that codes for apolipoprotein E, variant E4. Further work has shown that APOE ε4 has its predominant effect by determining when, but not if, a person develops late-onset Alzheimer's disease.[12] It seems though that possession of APOE ε4 is neither necessary, nor sufficient for disease initiation.

Non-genetic risk factors

Non-genetic risk factors are likely to be important in Alzheimer's disease as monozygotic twin concordance rates are only 40%.[13] Whilst much work has been carried out looking at the genetic risk factors, work to determine non-genetic risk factors has been slower.

The incidence and prevalence of Alzheimer's disease doubles every five years after 65 years of age. Age is therefore the single most important risk factor. At all ages, women are at an increased risk of developing Alzheimer's disease (the reverse of the situation with vascular dementia). This may be explained by hormonal factors. Some studies have suggested that oestrogen replacement can prevent or delay the onset of Alzheimer's disease. A 16-year follow-up of nearly 500 women found that hormone replacement therapy led to a 54% reduction in the risk of Alzheimer's disease.[14] A more recent trial was not able to demonstrate any improvement in cognition or disease progression in subjects with Alzheimer's given therapeutic oestrogen.[15]

Poor education has recently been cited as a risk factor for Alzheimer's disease, especially in males.[16] The concept of a protective effect of education has found some support.[17] However, it remains to be seen if it is childhood education that is protective, or whether it is the knowledge acquired over the lifetime.

Boxers experiencing repeated head trauma may develop dementia pugilistica. This is associated with pathological changes similar to those found in Alzheimer's disease. However, recent research has failed to implicate head trauma as a risk factor for Alzheimer's disease.[18] The relationship between Alzheimer's disease and aluminium is also unclear at present. Solvents and other heavy metals have not been shown to be risk factors.

Several studies have shown smoking to be protective against Alzheimer's disease. A confounding factor in these studies may be that those subjects who smoke, die before they reach an age at which Alzheimer's disease is prevalent. Other vascular risk factors such as hypertension and insulin-dependent diabetes have also been associated with Alzheimer's disease.[19]

Conflicting results have come from studies looking at the link between depression and dementia. Some suggest that depression is actually an early manifestation of dementia, whilst in other studies, depressive symptoms have been found to increase the risk of subsequent cognitive decline.[20]

Many studies have reported that the intake of NSAIDs is negatively associated with the risk of developing Alzheimer's disease. These findings should be interpreted with some caution. Patients with Alzheimer's may be less able to complain of pain and therefore receive treatment. These drugs may work by delaying nerve cell damage. This information is summarised in Box 3.1.

Box 3.1   Risk factors for Alzheimer's disease

Increased risk
- Increasing age
- Female sex

Possible increased risk
- Poor education
- Head trauma

Possible decreased risk
- Smoking
- NSAIDs

Evidence unclear at present
- Aluminium
- Depression

Vascular dementia

The term 'vascular dementia' literally means a dementia due to vascular disease. It encompasses a group of conditions, including multi-infarct dementia, subcortical dementia and Binswanger's subcortical arteriosclerotic encephalopathy. A diagnosis of vascular dementia requires the following *ICD-10* criteria[2] to be met:

- the general criteria for dementia
- deficits in higher cognitive function are unevenly distributed, with some functions affected and others relatively spared
- clinical evidence of focal brain damage, manifest in at least one of the following:
  - unilateral spastic weakness of the limbs
  - unilaterally increased tendon reflexes
  - an extended plantar response
  - pseudobulbar palsy
- evidence of a significant cerebrovascular disease, which may reasonably be judged to be aetiologically related to the dementia.

Clinical features

The onset is usually after the age of 65 and may follow a cerebral infarct. It may therefore present more acutely than Alzheimer's disease. Arteriosclerotic changes will often be found in the peripheral and retinal blood vessels, and the patient may well have hypertension. Emotional and personality changes may occur before any memory problems. Cognitive impairment tends to fluctuate in severity once it is established. The disease usually progresses in a stepwise manner, with periods of deterioration that are followed by stable periods or even periods of improvement. These more settled episodes might last for several months in the early stages. Insight may be maintained to a late stage. Other features can include:

- minor episodes of cerebral ischaemia (transient ischaemic attacks)
- depression (may be a result of retained insight) and anxiety
- episodes of emotional lability
- epileptic seizures (found in approximately 20% of cases).

The life span averages four to seven years from the time of diagnosis, though it may be much longer. Death may result from ischaemic heart disease, cerebral infarction or renal complications. There are a number of different subtypes of vascular dementia and a brief description of each is given below.

Multi-infarct dementia

This is a type of vascular dementia where the onset is gradual, following a number of ischaemic episodes. Each of these often leads to greater cognitive deficits. It may be caused by large-vessel disease and/or small-vessel disease. It is a predominantly cortical dementia.

Subcortical vascular dementia

In this type of dementia, the cerebral cortex is relatively spared. This contrasts with the clinical picture, which may closely resemble that of Alzheimer's dementia. The general criteria for vascular dementia must be met, as well as a history of hypertension and evidence of vascular disease in the deep white matter of the cerebral hemispheres, with preservation of the cerebral cortex.

Binswanger's disease

This is also known as progressive small-vessel disease or subcortical arteriosclerotic encephalopathy. It is a rare form of vascular dementia, first described by Binswanger in 1894.[21] Dementia may dominate the clinical picture but there may be concomitant physical problems, e.g. dysarthria and gait disorders. It is classically a slowly progressive dementia.

Cerebral autosomal dominant arteriopathy with subcortical infarcts and leukoencephalopthy (CADASIL)

A rare familial form of vascular dementia. Patients usually present in their forties with recurrent strokes. Quite often there is a history of migraine and many patients go on to develop a subcortical dementia and pseudobulbar palsy.

Other rare causes of vascular dementia

Cerebral vasculitis may cause repeated infarcts, and these may result in a dementia. The vasculitis usually involves many organs, resulting in other systemic features, e.g. systemic lupus erythematosus. Cognitive problems may also be noted after cerebral and extracerebral haemorrhages, often as a residual problem. Dementia may also occur as a result of multiple infarcts occurring during hypotensive crises, and as a result of chronic subdural haematomas.

The Hachinski score

Hachinski developed a scoring system which has been widely used as a guide to help clinicians distinguish between vascular dementia and Alzheimer's dementia.[22] The features are weighted as shown in Box 3.2. The scores of all features present are added together to give a total score, and a total score above six suggests a vascular dementia.

Box 3.2 The Hachinski ischaemia score

Abrupt onset	2
Stepwise deterioration	1
Fluctuating course	2
Nocturnal confusion	1
Relative preservation of personality	1
Depression	1
Somatic complaints	1
Emotional incontinence	1
History of hypertension	1
History of strokes	2
Atherosclerosis	2
Focal neurological symptoms	2
Focal neurological signs	2

Differentiating between vascular dementia and Alzheimer's dementia

Characteristically, Alzheimer's disease has an insidious onset and progresses slowly without any evidence of focal brain damage. In contrast, vascular dementia tends to present more acutely and progress in a stepwise manner. Findings compatible with ischaemic brain changes are also present. At times it is therefore clearly possible to differentiate the two types of dementia. At other times though it can be quite the opposite. Brain imaging techniques may be used to help in the diagnosis, e.g. to identify cerebral infarcts. As mentioned above, the Hachinski score is also used to assist in the diagnosis. However, sometimes the diagnosis can only be confirmed at post-mortem. It must also be remembered that a mixed vascular and Alzheimer's dementia is not uncommon.[23]

Risk factors for vascular dementia

The incidence of vascular dementia in men and women is almost equal, but it is slightly more common in men. There is considerable evidence to suggest that raised blood pressure earlier in life is a risk factor for dementia in later life. Research has shown that hypertension is the most important remedial risk factor for stroke and vascular dementia.[24] Work is ongoing at present to assess the effectiveness of antihypertensives in vascular dementia. Advancing age is a risk factor for stroke, and therefore also for vascular dementia.

Several studies have reported an increased incidence of dementia after strokes. However, not all cases of vascular dementia can be explained by the sequelae of stroke, ischaemia or hypoxia.

Cerebral white matter lesions are seen more frequently in patients with vascular dementia than in normal elderly subjects or patients with other dementias.

They have been shown to be predictors of post-stroke dementia.[25] A history of myocardial infarction is also a risk factor for vascular dementia as are atrial fibrillation, rheumatic valvular disease and carotid artery stenosis. Diabetes is a risk factor for vascular disease as it is associated with a reduction in cerebral perfusion, which may result in infarctions.[26]

Raised levels of low-density lipoproteins, in particular, have been shown to be a risk factor for the development of dementia with stroke. This relationship has not been found with Alzheimer's disease.[27]

Smoking has been shown to be a risk factor for vascular dementia by some,[28] but these results have not always been replicated. As with Alzheimer's dementia, a possible explanation could be that those who smoke have reduced life spans, and may die before developing a dementia. Many studies have shown an increased risk of vascular dementia in people with a history of alcohol misuse,[24] but not all studies have found this.[28]

There are many rare genetic disorders that are associated with stroke and subsequent vascular dementia. An increased risk of stroke or coronary heart disease has also been shown in patients with the APOE polymorphism. As previously stated, this is a risk factor for Alzheimer's disease. It is important to note here that many patients with Alzheimer's disease also have vascular changes, and one-fifth have been shown to have vascular lesions.[24] It is likely that the co-existing vascular problems in these patients will contribute to their cognitive decline.

Poor formal education has been associated with an increased risk of vascular dementia,[24] as have psychological stress in early life and 'blue-collar' occupations.[29] The Canadian Study of Health and Ageing showed elevated odds ratios for vascular dementia in people who had occupational exposure to pesticides, fertilisers, liquid plastics and rubbers.[24] This information is summarised in Box 3.3.

Box 3.3 Risk factors for vascular dementia

Increased risk
- Male sex
- Increasing age
- Hypertension
- Diabetes mellitus
- Previous stroke
- Cardiovascular disease
- High levels of low-density lipoproteins

Possible increased risk
- Smoking
- Alcohol misuse
- Poor education
- 'Blue collar' occupations
- Psychological stress in early life
- Previous exposure to pesticides, fertilisers, etc.

In order to reduce the risk of both stroke and vascular dementia, it is important that these risk factors are identified and treated as early as possible. Some cases of vascular dementia could be prevented (see Case Study 3.2).

Case Study 3.2

A 78-year-old gentleman went to see his GP with his wife. Over the last few months he had noticed that he had become increasingly forgetful, and his wife confirmed this. He was concerned that he may have Alzheimer's disease. The problems seemed to come on quite suddenly and since that time he reported episodes when he felt that his memory was awful, but other times when it was fairly good. He had mislaid items around the house and had put teabags in the kettle on a few occasions when making a cup of tea. His wife had also had to help him with their finances, as he no longer felt able to do this himself. He often had difficulty remembering the names of his children. There was no past psychiatric history but the patient was on treatment for hypertension and angina. He also smoked 20 cigarettes a day and had done so for 50 years. He did have some problems with his memory and concentration when the GP tested him. The GP requested a CT scan, which showed some brain atrophy and evidence of old infarctions. A diagnosis of a vascular dementia was made by the GP.

Lewy body dementia

Lewy bodies are the pathological hallmark of Parkinson's disease. However, they have also been found to occur in the cerebral cortex in association with dementia. Lewy body dementia is a common form of dementia in old age. Many patients with Lewy body dementia also show some Alzheimer-type changes, and minor vascular disease occurs in approximately 30%, i.e. mixed pathological changes are usually seen.[30]

Clinical features

Dementia is usually the presenting feature. However, patients may present with Parkinsonism, psychiatric disorder in the absence of dementia, falls, orthostatic hypotension or transient disturbances of consciousness.[31] The age at onset ranges from 50 to 83 years. Survival time from diagnosis is similar to that for Alzheimer's disease, but some patients do show a rapid progression of symptoms and death may occur within one to two years in these cases. The cognitive function seems to decline at a similar rate to that in Alzheimer's disease. It is slightly more common in men than women. Clinical features include:

- fluctuation in cognitive performance and level of consciousness (usually evident day to day), with pronounced variations in attention and alertness

- visual hallucinations (reported by approximately two-thirds of patients) – these are usually well formed and detailed

- depression (occurs in 40%)

- parkinsonism (occurs in up to 70% of patients, e.g. bradykinesia, limb rigidity and gait disturbances)

- repeated falls and syncope.

Other features that may support the diagnosis are sensitivity to neuroleptic medication (found in up to 50% of patients), systematised delusions and hallucinations in other modalities. Lewy body dementia is a fairly new concept and is not defined within *ICD-10*, but consensus criteria for the clinical diagnosis of probable and possible dementia with Lewy bodies have been put forward.[32] These include the features mentioned above and also state that a diagnosis of Lewy body dementia is less likely in the presence of stroke disease, or if there is evidence of any physical illness or other brain disorder which could account for the clinical picture. The diagnostic accuracy has not yet been established outside of specialist research settings and this is an area for further work. There is also a grey area between the diagnoses of Lewy body dementia and Parkinson's disease with dementia or psychosis. Should these all be classified as a 'Lewy body disease spectrum' or should they remain as separate categories? The debate is ongoing.

There is obviously much more work to be done within the field of Lewy body dementia, especially with regard to establishing diagnostic accuracy in the community and defining aetiological factors. Research is also currently ongoing to find effective treatments for Lewy body dementia.

Depressive pseudodementia

An elderly person may present with reduced interests, psychomotor retardation, slowed thinking and concentration, poor short-term memory and disorientation. This readily mimics dementia when actually there is an underlying depression, hence the term depressive pseudodementia. However, it must be remembered that depression frequently occurs in the early stages of dementia, so the diagnosis may be difficult. When the situation is unclear, a careful history and mental state should help to differentiate the two. Points to consider are:

- onset – more likely to be acute in depression and insidious in dementia

- memory decline prior to the current episode – less likely in depression than in dementia

- observations from a close family member

- is the patient distressed by the situation? Patients with depression will often complain of their difficulties, unlike patients with dementia

- responses to questions – a tendency in depressed patients to reply, 'Don't know', whereas a patient with dementia may confabulate or make excuses for not knowing
- any family history of depression or dementia?
- are symptoms of depression present?
- performance on cognitive function tests – may be inconsistent in depression, where inattention is often the main problem and dysphasia and dyspraxia will be absent.

These points may help when trying to differentiate between depression and dementia.

Delirium superimposed on dementia

Patients with dementia may also present as acutely confused at times. This is often described as an acute on chronic confusion or as a delirium superimposed on dementia. The definition of delirium in *ICD-10*[2] is as follows:

- there is clouding of consciousness
- disturbance of cognition is manifest by impairment of immediate recall and recent memory (with relatively intact remote memory), and also disorientation in time, place or person
- At least one of:
  - rapid unpredictable shifts from hypoactivity to hyperactivity
  - increased reaction time
  - increased or decreased flow of speech
  - enhanced startle reaction
- disturbance of sleep or the sleep–wake cycle, causing insomnia and/or nocturnal worsening of symptoms and/or disturbing dreams and nightmares
- symptoms have a rapid onset and fluctuate over the course of the day
- obvious evidence of an underlying cerebral or systemic disease that can be presumed to be responsible for the clinical manifestations.

Almost any acute illness can cause a delirium in an elderly person. The most common causes are urinary tract infections, chest infections, cardiac failure and iatrogenic causes.

Dementia is a risk factor for delirium; indeed, it has been identified as one of three major risk factors for delirium.[33] Other predisposing factors include:[34]

- ageing or disease of the brain
- impairment of vision and hearing

- reduced synthesis of neurotransmitters
- changes in pharmacokinetics and dynamics of drugs
- high prevalence of chronic diseases
- high susceptibility to acute diseases
- reduced capacity for homeostatic regulation.

A thorough history with a mental state examination, a physical examination and appropriate investigations should help to determine the cause. The appropriate specific treatment can then be administered, along with supportive care. This is most often undertaken in a general hospital.

Key points

- Dementia is a syndrome with a number of different causes.
- It is usually more common with increasing age, progressive and irreversible.
- The most common types of dementia are Alzheimer's disease, vascular dementia and Lewy body dementia.
- Defining the cause of the dementia will inform decisions on treatment and prognosis.
- Diagnostic criteria for dementia can be found in *DSM-IV* and *ICD-10*.
- A full history, mental state examination, physical examination and further investigations, e.g. blood tests and CT scans, should help to clarify the cause of the dementia.
- Alzheimer's disease is the most common cause of dementia. It tends to progress gradually through three clinical stages.
- Whilst an autosomal dominant pattern has been described in several cases of Alzheimer's disease starting before 65 years of age, this is extremely rare in those cases starting after 65 years.
- Several non-genetic risk factors for Alzheimer's disease have been proposed.
- Vascular dementia may present acutely and characteristically progresses in a stepwise manner.
- Many of the risk factors for vascular dementia are the same as those for cardiovascular disease. Early identification and treatment of these risk factors could therefore potentially prevent some cases of vascular dementia.
- Lewy body dementia has been described more recently and consensus criteria for its diagnosis have been proposed which describe the clinical features.
- Mixed patterns of dementia, such as mixed Alzheimer's and vascular dementia, are not uncommon.
- Depressive pseudodementia and delirium superimposed on dementia should be considered when a patient presents with a possible diagnosis of dementia.

References

1 Lishman WA (1987) *Organic Psychiatry.* Blackwell Science, Oxford.
2 World Health Organization (1992) *The ICD-10 Classification of Mental and Behavioural Disorders: clinical descriptions and diagnostic guidelines.* WHO, Geneva.
3 McArthur JC, Hoover DR, Bacellar H *et al.* (1993) Dementia in AIDS patients: incidence and risk factors. *Neurology.* **43**: 2245–52.
4 Edwards G (1982) *The Treatment of Drinking Problems.* Grant McIntyre, London.
5 Cummings JL (1986) Subcortical dementia. Neuropsychology, neuropsychiatry and pathophysiology. *British Journal of Psychiatry.* **149**: 682–97.
6 American Psychiatric Association (1994) *Diagnostic and Statistical Manual of Mental Disorders* (4e). APA, Washington DC.
7 Alzheimer A (1907) Uber eine eigenartige Erkrankung der Hirnrinde. *Allgemeine Zeitschrift fur Psychiatrie und Psychisch-Gerichtlich Medizin.* **64**: 146–8.
8 Gao S, Hendrie HC, Hall KS *et al.* (1998) The relationships between age, sex and the incidence of dementia and Alzheimer disease: a meta-analysis. *Archives of General Psychiatry.* **55**: 809–15.
9 Hughes CP, Berg L, Danziger W *et al.* (1982) A new clinical scale for the staging of dementia. *British Journal of Psychiatry.* **140**: 566–72.
10 Reisberg B, Ferris S, De Leon MJ *et al.* (1982) The Global Deterioration Scale (GDS): an instrument for the assessment of primary degenerative dementia. *American Journal of Psychiatry.* **139**: 1136–9.
11 Cruts M, van Duijn CM, Backhovens H *et al.* (1998) Estimation of the genetic contribution of presenilin-1 and -2 mutations in a population based study of presenile Alzheimer's disease. *Human Molecular Genetics.* **7**: 43–51.
12 Meyer MR, Tschanz JT, Norton MC *et al.* (1998) APOE genotype predicts when – not whether – one is predisposed to develop Alzheimer's disease. *Nature Genetics.* **19**: 321–2.
13 Pericak-Vance MA and Haines JL (1995) Genetic susceptibility to Alzheimer's disease. *Trends in Genetics.* **11**: 504–8.
14 Kawas C, Resnick S, Morrison A *et al.* (1997) A prospective study of estrogen replacement therapy and the risk of developing Alzheimer's disease: the Baltimore Longitudinal Study of Aging. *Neurology.* **48**: 1517–21.
15 Mulnard RA, Cotman CW, Kawas C *et al.* (2000) Estrogen replacement therapy for treatment of mild to moderate Alzheimer's disease: a randomised controlled trial. Alzheimer's Disease Cooperative Study. *Journal of the American Medical Association.* **283**: 1007–15.
16 Ott A, van Rossum CT, van Harskamp F *et al.* (1999) Education and the incidence of dementia in a large population-based study: the Rotterdam Study. *Neurology.* **52**: 663–6.
17 Orrell M and Sahakian B (1995) Education and dementia. *British Medical Journal.* **310**: 951–2.
18 Launer LJ, Andersen K, Dewey ME *et al.* (1999) Rates and risk factors for dementia and Alzheimer's disease: results from EURODEM pooled analyses.

EURODEM Incidence Research Group and Work Groups – European studies of dementia. *Neurology*. **52**: 78–84.

19 Stewart R, Prince M and Mann A (1999) Vascular risk factors and Alzheimer's disease. *Australian and New Zealand Journal of Psychiatry*. **33**: 809–13.

20 Yaffe K, Blackwell T, Gore R *et al.* (1999) Depressive symptoms and cognitive decline in nondemented elderly women: a prospective study. *Archives of General Psychiatry*. **56**: 425–30.

21 Binswanger O (1894) Die Abgrenzung der allgemeinen progressiven paralyse. *Berliner klinische Wochenshrift*. **31**: 1137–9.

22 Hachinski VC, Lliff LD, Kilhka M *et al.* (1975) Cerebral blood flow in dementia. *Archives of Neurology*. **32**: 632–7.

23 Jellinger K, Danielczyk W, Fischer P *et al.* (1990) Clinicopathological analysis of dementia disorders in the elderly. *Journal of Neurological Sciences*. **95**: 239–58.

24 Lindsay J, Hebert R and Rockwood K (1997) The Canadian Study of Health and Aging: risk factors for vascular dementia. *Stroke*. **28**: 526–30.

25 Miyos S, Takano A, Teramoto J *et al.* (1992) Leukoariosis in relation to prognosis for patients with lacunar infarction. *Stroke*. **233**: 1434–8.

26 Desmond DW, Tatemichi TK, Paik M *et al.* (1993) Risk factors for cerebrovascular disease as correlates of cognitive function in a stroke-free cohort. *Archives of Neurology*. **50**: 162–6.

27 Moroney JT, Tang MX, Bergkind L *et al.* (1999) Low-density lipoprotein cholesterol and the risk of dementia with stroke. *Journal of the American Medical Association*. **282**: 254–60.

28 Meyer JS, McClintik K, Rogers RL *et al.* (1988) Aetiological considerations and risk factors for multi-infarct dementia. *Journal of Neurology and Neurosurgical Psychiatry*. **51**: 1489–97.

29 Peerson G and Skoog I (1996) A prospective population study of psychosocial risk factors for late-onset dementia. *International Journal of Geriatric Psychiatry*. **11**: 15–22.

30 Holmes C, Cairns N, Lantos P *et al.* (1999) Validity of current clinical criteria for Alzheimer's disease, vascular dementia and dementia with Lewy bodies. *British Journal of Psychiatry*. **174**: 45–50.

31 McKeith IG, Perry RH, Fairbairn AF *et al.* (1992) Operational criteria for senile dementia of Lewy body type (SDLT). *Psychological Medicine*. **22**: 911–22.

32 McKeith IG, Galasko D, Kosaka K *et al.* (1996) Consensus guidelines for the clinical and pathologic diagnosis of dementia with Lewy bodies (DLB): report of the consortium on DLB international workshop. *Neurology*. **47**: 1113–24.

33 O'Keefe S and Lavan J (1996) Predicting delirium in elderly patients: development and validation of a risk-stratification model. *Age and Ageing*. **25**: 317–21.

34 Lipowski ZJ (1987) Delirium (acute confusional states). *Journal of the American Geriatrics Society*. **258**: 1789–92.

4

Early detection of dementia

Loopinder Sood, John P Wattis and Stephen Curran

Introduction

In Alzheimer's disease (AD) and other forms of dementia, irreversible brain damage usually occurs before clinical symptoms become apparent. Drugs for the treatment of mild to moderate AD are now available and the sooner such drugs can be given, the greater the potential clinical benefit. This has led to a drive to try and detect AD at an early stage, ideally before memory disturbance becomes apparent. There is therefore a pressing need for an easy to use and inexpensive means of screening people at risk of developing AD which would help to diagnose AD at an early stage. Other forms of dementia also need to be identified early so that further decline can be halted or symptoms reversed. Tests which are used as screening instruments are generally quick and easy to use and help to identify potential cases of AD. These cases can then be examined in greater detail using a variety of techniques to establish the diagnosis. In addition, a number of tests may be potentially useful as screening instruments, such as neuroimaging techniques, but because of cost or practical considerations would only be suitable in a research context.

Risks and benefits of early detection

The early detection of dementia is important for a number of reasons. Firstly, early diagnosis will give patients an opportunity to discuss their symptoms, treatment options and prognosis and make informed choices about their future. Patients will be able to plan for the future and make their wishes known about residential care and other issues, such as setting up an Enduring Power of Attorney. Families can also be supported at a much earlier stage and crises can be minimised or avoided. Patients with reversible causes for their cognitive impairment, e.g. vitamin B_{12} deficiency, can be treated (see Table 4.1) and symptoms frequently reversed. Patients with vascular dementia can stabilise their symptoms in part by improving their physical health and a number of lifestyle changes such as stopping smoking, eating a healthier diet, doing more exercise and paying more attention to their physical health. In addition, lifestyle changes geared to improvements in cardiovascular health could also impact on the onset of AD, since risk factors for cerebrovascular disease are also risk factors for dementia, including AD.[1] Hence, interventions that modify vascular risk factors might also be able to delay the onset of AD or slow its rate of progression. In addition, drugs for the treatment of AD are more likely to be effective if they are given early, though paradoxically the effects at this stage may be less obvious.[2] From the research point of view, early and accurate detection and diagnosis are important in allowing assessment of the efficacy of interventions at a stage when they are likely to be most effective.

Early detection is therefore important as it:

• gives patients a greater say in their future care

• helps patients and their families to plan for the future

• may enhance the effectiveness of medication

• enables research into the efficacy of early intervention.

However, not all the consequences of early detection are necessarily positive. The diagnosis will be stressful for patients and carers and because the natural history of dementia is well known, this can be an alarming diagnosis, and can result in a range of psychological reactions including 'shock and bewilderment' initially and subsequently followed by a range of emotions including anger, depression and denial. However a particular patient and their family copes with the diagnosis, it is nearly always stressful and it has a dramatic impact on their lives and future plans. If the diagnosis subsequently turns out to be wrong, the consequences can be devastating and patients and their families will feel very angry. If possible, pre- and post-diagnostic counselling should be available, but this is rarely the case. In the early stages, overlap with healthy ageing and depression is common and a balance needs to be struck between early diagnosis and getting the diagnosis correct. There is currently no diagnostic test for many of the different kinds of dementia and AD in particular, but as the condition progresses accurate diagnosis usually becomes easier.

Characteristics of diagnostic and screening tests

There is considerable overlap between screening and diagnostic tests and to some extent they have similar characteristics. A *screening* instrument needs to be relatively simple to use. It is usually administered to large groups of people and those patients identified are then subjected to more intensive investigation. Screening instruments have a number of desirable characteristics. Some of these are practical in nature, some cost-related and some methodological. Screening instruments should be easy to administer for both the tester and patient. They should be relatively quick, safe and cheap to administer and should not cause undue anxiety for the patient. They should also be portable and require minimal training. They should be valid (measure what the test is supposed to measure, such as cognitive function) and reliable. The latter requirement can be split into test–retest reliability (are the results the same on two separate occasions?) and inter-rater reliability (are the results the same when the test is administered by two different people?). Screening instruments usually identify patients who are more likely to have a disorder but require further investigation, e.g. patients who score poorly on the Mini-Mental State Examination (MMSE) test which might be due to a number of factors. Further questioning and examination might lead to a diagnosis of AD, but the MMSE is not a diagnostic test – what is detected (cognitive impairment) is not specific to dementia. For this reason, additional assessment is needed to make the diagnosis. In this sense most of the so-called 'diagnostic' tests are really screening tests.

Tests should also be sensitive and specific. The sensitivity is the ability of the test to *correctly detect the condition*, and is the proportion of people with the condition who test positive. The specificity is the ability of the test to *correctly identify subjects who do not have the condition*, and is the proportion of people without the condition who test negative. The ideal test should correctly identify all subjects with the condition, as well as all subjects without, and would have a sensitivity and specificity both equal to 100%. Tests that make 'mistakes' are less than ideal and miss the condition in some subjects who do have it and/or identify the condition in some subjects who do not have it. The concept of sensitivity and specificity is summarised in Table 4.1. The sensitivity is a/(a+c) whereas the specificity is d/(b+d).[3] Some of the other commonly used terms include *positive predictive value* (PPV); if the test is positive, the PPV is the probability that the patient has the condition [a/a+b] and *negative predictive value* (NPP); if the test is negative, the NPP is the probability that the patient does not have the condition [d/c+d].

Table 4.1 Table for calculating sensitivity and specificity

	Disease present	Disease absent
Test positive	a	b
Test negative	c	d

a = true positives, b = false positives, c = false negatives and d = true negatives.
In an ideal test, b = c = 0.

Potential screening tests can be classified into a number of groups, including clinical assessment, rating scales, other psychometric tests, neuroimaging techniques, biochemical tests, biopsy and genetic tests. Although there is considerable overlap between screening and diagnostic tests, these have been separated for convenience. Screening tests are usually not diagnostic but are used to identify patients at high risk of having a particular condition such as AD. These patients can then undergo a fuller diagnostic evaluation. The situation is further confused by simple tests that can be used in the community and those that tend either to be confined to specialist centres or are not widely available because they are still undergoing evaluation.

Diagnostic tests

Clinical assessment

This is an important part of the diagnostic process and should include a detailed history, mental state examination, physical examination and information should be obtained from other sources, especially carers. The nature of the memory impairment as well as its course, duration and associated features, such as focal signs, should be evaluated. Previous psychiatric history, family history of memory impairment and current medication can also be very helpful. In addition, many drugs, especially psychiatric drugs, can cause confusion and memory impairment. The patient's medical history is also important as this might point to a specific cause and examples include cerebrovascular disease, head injury and vitamin B_{12} deficiency. Additional aspects of the history that should be asked about include previous occupation, activities of daily living, the presence of psychiatric symptoms such as depression and psychotic symptoms, and any carer stress. This information combined with further investigations will help to establish the diagnosis. As well as identifying a specific cause of the dementia, they will also identify any potentially reversible cause for the dementia (see Box 4.1) and any psychiatric syndromes, such as depression, anxiety or psychotic phenomena, that will require treatment in their own right. Attention to these will improve not only the quality of life for patients with cognitive impairment but also in some cases reduce their mortality, particularly in the case of depression.

A detailed physical examination is also an important part of the diagnostic process in dementia and this combined with other information should then result in the patient undergoing a more detailed psychiatric assessment. From a practical perspective, the GP is probably in the best position to comment on the physical health of the patient, and where this is unclear a local protocol should be developed to clarify the roles of the different healthcare professionals to make the patient's journey as smooth as possible and to avoid unnecessary duplication of work and investigations.

Following the psychiatric and medical history and physical examination, a number of investigations such as kidney, liver, thyroid and other blood tests can be undertaken, and additional investigation as indicated such as ECGs, chest X-rays and neuroimaging techniques (see below), to clarify the diagnosis and help to identify any potentially reversible case for the cognitive impairment (see Box 4.1). For a more detailed examination of the physical aspects of dementia, see Chapter 7.

Neuroimaging

Although in theory neuroimaging could be used in screening programmes, in practice its cost means it is more useful for research purposes or for confirming the diagnosis in patients already shown to have cognitive impairment.

Box 4.1   Some causes of reversible dementia

Intracranial
- Subdural haematoma
- Tumour
- Abscess

Central nervous system infection
- Syphilis
- Tuberculosis
- Fungal infections

Endocrine
- Hyper/hypothyroidism
- Hyper/hypoparathyroidism
- Hyper/hypoadrenalism

Collagen diseases
- Systemic lupus erythematosus
- Temporal arteritis

Metabolic
- Liver disease
- Renal disease
- Wilson's disease
- Pernicious anaemia
- Folate deficiency

Toxic
- Alcohol
- Heavy metals, e.g. aluminium

Psychiatric
- Depression/mania
- Schizophrenia
- Conversion disorder
- Ganser syndrome

Miscellaneous
- Communicating hydrocephalus
- Epilepsy
- Parkinson's disease
- Remote effect of various cancers
- Cardiac insufficiency
- Respiratory insufficiency

Structural neuroimaging

Structural neuroimaging is useful in the diagnostic work-up for patients with dementia, helping to exclude potentially reversible causes of dementia. Magnetic resonance imaging (MRI) in AD has shown that entorhinal cortex volumetry and also hippocampal volumetry can discriminate between those with mild cognitive deficits and healthy controls.[4] Longitudinal studies of AD have shown that general brain atrophy in terms of total brain volume determined by serial MRI is in the range of 1–2.8% per year for AD, much larger than the rate of 0.05–0.41% per year for elderly controls.[4] Patients with AD also had accelerated rate of hippocampal atrophy compared with controls. Thus MRI could be used alongside clinical assessment to detect early AD.[5] However, MRI is an expensive procedure and it is not readily available, especially for large-scale screening of community-based patients.

A recent CT scan study examined medial temporal lobe atrophy in ten patients with mild cognitive impairment, 42 patients with AD and 29 non-demented controls. When the specificity was fixed at 95%, the sensitivity for AD was found to be 93% and for mild cognitive impairment 80%.[6]

Functional imaging

Magnetic resonance spectroscopy (MRS) has also been suggested as a useful technique for the early detection of AD. MRS is an imaging technique that can determine the amount of cerebral metabolites in the living brain, including N-acetylaspartate (NAA), choline-containing compounds (Cho), creatine-phosphocreatine (Cr) and myoinositol (MI). NAA is considered to be a neurone marker and has been extensively studied in AD, and reductions in its concentration have been found in the brains of patients with AD. MI is considered to be a tentative glial marker and to represent gliosis severity in AD.[4] It has been suggested that the severity of AD can be monitored by the relative reduction of NAA/Cr concentration ratio in the medial temporal lobe. MRS findings in other dementias have been compared with AD. On the basis of MI elevation being larger in frontotemporal dementia compared with AD, 92% of patients with frontotemporal dementia were correctly differentiated from AD. Small studies of MRS comparing AD with vascular dementia have suggested regional differences in disease distribution, with more involvement of the frontal lobe in vascular dementia and the parietal lobe in AD. It has also been found that patients with vascular dementia had lower NAA/Cr and NAA/Cho ratios in the subcortical white matter compared with patients with AD. These findings need confirmation in larger studies. In addition, MRS is not practical in clinical practice due to limited availability and poor spatial resolution.

Other studies have suggested that photon emission tomography (PET) scans might be helpful. Recent findings suggest that in patients with AD, changes in the posterior cingulate, temporoparietal and prefrontal association cortex correlated with dementia severity. In patients with mild to moderate AD, the sensitivity and specificity were 93%. This fell to 84% sensitivity and 93% specificity for patients with MMSE scores ≥ 24.[7]

Another technique that has been investigated involves examining activated microglia. These have a key role in the brain's immune response to neuronal degeneration. This is associated with an increased expression of receptors known as peripheral benzodiazepine binding sites. Using PET techniques (Carbon-11-labelled R-PK11195), binding properties have been shown not to change with age, but there is significantly increased binding in patients with mild AD, particularly in the entorhinal, temporoparietal and cingulate cortex.[8]

However, structural and functional neuroimaging techniques are relatively expensive, cumbersome and generally confined to specialist centres. Although they are helpful to rule out specific causes of dementia such as tumours, stroke disease, etc., there is considerable overlap with healthy ageing, and they are not particularly helpful for the early diagnosis of AD and it is unlikely that they would ever be used as a screening instrument for large numbers of community-based patients with mild or pre-clinical cognitive impairment.

Biochemical tests

A number of neurological conditions clinically similar to AD are caused by transmissible agents. These include kuru, Creutzfeldt–Jakob disease and Gerstmann–Straussler syndrome. These diseases are due to prions which, until relatively recently, were unknown infectious agents. Prions have a long incubation period with none of the inflammatory responses seen with viral infections. This raises the possibility that AD might also be caused by a transmissible agent, but evidence remains unconvincing. However, the only biochemical test that has become established in clinical practice is the measurement of the protein 14-3-3 in cerebrospinal fluid to help diagnose sporadic cases of Creutzfeldt–Jakob disease.

Diagnostic schedules

AD, one of the common causes of dementia, can be diagnosed with high sensitivity (85%) using standardised criteria.[9] A number of diagnostic schedules are also frequently used in clinical practice, including *DSM-IV*[10] and *ICD-10*,[11] and these are discussed more fully in Chapter 3.

Screening tests

Tests for cognitive impairment

One of the most widely used cognitive tests is the Mini-Mental State Examination.[12] It has a high sensitivity and specificity (87%) for dementia in older people with memory impairment. It is a short cognitive test, which takes about ten minutes or less to administer, it is not stressful for patients and can easily be incorporated into clinical practice with a minimal amount of training. It is a screening instrument and should not be used as a diagnostic test. Patients who have evidence of cognitive impairment need to be further evaluated, partly to establish the diagnosis of dementia and then to clarify the specific cause of the dementia.

The clock-drawing test is also clinically useful, takes only a few minutes to perform and has a sensitivity and specificity of 85% for dementia with good inter-rater reliability.[13] It taps into a wide range of cognitive abilities and is also able to detect deterioration, but cannot distinguish between the different causes of dementia. However, it is useful when language is a barrier to cognitive testing, but caution needs to be exercised when used in patients with low educational achievement.

The six-item Cognitive Impairment Test (6CIT) is an improvement on the MMSE as it is quicker to administer and outperforms it in milder dementia.[14] It should therefore prove to be a better screening tool than the MMSE for identifying milder cases of dementia which the MMSE would miss, but further work is needed to establish this.

The early detection of dementia might also be aided by a screening test which could be administered by the family. The Symptoms of Dementia Screener (SDS) is an 11-item questionnaire, designed for use by lay persons, and can also be administered over the telephone.[15] A score of five or more is associated with a sensitivity of 90.2% and a specificity of 84.6% for dementia in community-based samples of patients with cognitive impairment.

Tests for Alzheimer's disease

In an attempt to improve the usefulness of the MMSE, one retrospective pragmatic study set in a district general old age psychiatric service investigated whether the spread of scores on the seven subsections of the MMSE, rather than the total score, could be used to classify dementia into Alzheimer's dementia and non-Alzheimer's dementia.

Case notes of those patients with cognitive decline were identified from discharge records and also by contacting the community psychiatric nurses. MMSE scores in each of the seven subsections (orientation, registration, attention, recall, language, three-stage command, pentagon construction), total scores and the clinical diagnosis made by the consultant were recorded. There were a total of 45 cases with dementia, 14 AD and 31 non-AD. The results showed that it was not possible to classify dementia into AD and non-AD based on the spread of scores on the seven subsections of the MMSE (Sood, 2003, unpublished).

The Cambridge Cognitive Examination (CAMCOG), a screening instrument, was evaluated in a dataset comprising healthy subjects, subjects with incident AD and subjects with prevalent AD to investigate its ability to detect early AD.[16] The authors concluded that for the early detection of AD it was best to use the memory and non-memory scores of the test separately instead of the total score, since it was found that a low memory score in the context of a relatively good general cognition predicted early stages of AD. However, whilst this study confirmed the clinical experience that memory problems arise early in AD, it did not investigate whether the CAMCOG instrument could be used to distinguish AD from other dementias. Neither did the study establish whether the instrument could pick out AD from patients presenting to clinical practice with cognitive problems.

More recently, two subtests (paired associate learning and delayed matching) of the Cambridge Neuropsychological Test Automated Battery (CANTAB) identified all cases of early AD that subsequently met diagnostic criteria for AD.[17]

Semenza et al.[18] also compared the efficiency of three instruments at distinguishing subjects with AD from healthy controls. Two tests requiring proper name retrieval were prepared and compared against the MMSE[12] and the Modified MMSE (3MS).[19] It was found that the MMSE had a ceiling effect and was not able to detect milder cases of AD from the control group. The 3MS was more sensitive than the MMSE due to its 'verbal fluency subtest' and the proper name retrieval test was more sensitive still.

Other studies did attempt to distinguish AD from other types of dementia. Mathuranath et al.[20] validated a simple bedside test battery (Addenbrooke's Cognitive Examination, ACE), designed to detect mild dementia and differentiate AD from frontotemporal dementia. The ACE is a 100-point test battery, assessing six cognitive areas – orientation, attention, memory, verbal fluency, language and visuospatial ability – and takes 15–20 minutes to administer. Patients with dementia were compared with a control group. It was found that the ACE had a higher sensitivity than the MMSE for the early detection of dementia and it could differentiate AD from frontotemporal dementia in mildly demented patients. Some of these tests are summarised in Table 4.2.

Table 4.2 Pencil and paper tests for detecting dementia

	MMSE	6CIT	SDS	CAMCOG	CANTAB	ACE
Low cost	+	+	+	+/-	+/-	+/-
Ease of use	+	+	+	+/-	+/-	+/-
Portable	+	+	+	+	+/-	+
Low risk	+	+	+	+	+	+
Detection of dementia	+/-	+	+	+	+	+
Detection of type of dementia	-	-	-	-	-	+/-
Established reliability	+/-	+	+	+	+	+
Useful in mild dementia	-	+	+/-	+	+	+
Useful in pre-clinical dementia	-	-	-	-	-	-

MMSE, Mini Mental State Examination test; 6CIT, six-item Cognitive Impairment Test; SDS, Symptoms of Dementia Screener; CAMCOG, Cambridge Cognitive Examination; CANTAB, Cambridge Neuropsychological Test Automated Battery; ACE, Addenbrooke's Cognitive Examination.

Other psychometric tests

Critical Flicker Fusion Threshold (CFFT)

Critical Flicker Fusion Threshold is a well-established neurophysiological technique which has been extensively studied in young and older healthy volunteers.

The neurophysiological basis of flicker perception is well described.[21] Flickering light directly influences cortical activity (measured by electroencephalogram, EEG), and although flickering light is able to initiate neuronal activity in various parts of the visual system (from retina to cortex), the temporal resolution of CFFT appears to be determined principally by the occipital cortex. Above a particular frequency, flickering light does not appear to flicker, and the point at which this occurs is the CFFT and is a measure of the information-processing capacity of the central nervous system. In the ascending mode, the frequency of flicker is gradually increased until the flickering lights appear to stop flickering – this is the ascending threshold. In the descending mode, the frequency of flicker is gradually decreased until the lights appear to start flickering – this is the descending threshold. The CFFT is the average of the ascending and descending thresholds.

   CFFT has been examined in a large community sample of healthy older people (n = 644) and scores were normally distributed. Descending thresholds were significantly higher than ascending thresholds, confirming findings from studies in younger subjects. In addition, there were no significant correlations between CFFT, ascending and descending thresholds and age. However, although not significant, there was a negative correlation between age and descending thresholds. The lack of a correlation between CFFT, ascending and descending thresholds and age is important since if CFFT were correlated with age, this measure would probably be unable to distinguish change in cognitive function due to age or the disease process in a longitudinal context, e.g. as a screening instrument. In a further study, CFFT and ascending and descending thresholds were examined in patients with AD and healthy controls. CFFT and descending thresholds were significantly lower in patients with AD compared with healthy controls, whereas ascending thresholds were not significantly different in the two groups. In addition, in the patient group, ascending thresholds were also significantly higher than descending thresholds: this latter finding is a reversal of the situation seen in healthy older subjects and this might be a characteristic feature of AD. In a series of further studies in patients with AD, CFFT has also been shown to have a high test–retest reliability, high inter-rater reliability and to be a valid measure in patients with AD. These studies have been described elsewhere in more detail.[21] CFFT is quick and easy to administer as well as being cheap and portable. It requires relatively little training and has high validity and reliability in patients with AD, and would be suitable to evaluate further as a screening test.

Choice Reaction Time (CRT)

Choice Reaction Time is a widely used measure with an extensive body of literature. Hindmarch and Wattis[22] have suggested that CRT is an indicator of sensori-motor performance, a common feature of many 'everyday' activities. It has also been proposed as a measure of the efficiency of attentional and response mechanisms in the information-processing chain, without the need for extensive cognitive processing.[23] In this test, subjects are required to respond to a critical stimulus, and the time taken to do this is recorded. However, because the subject is presented with a number of identical stimuli, this also provides a measure of attentional monitoring abilities. A number of studies have demonstrated significant reductions in reaction times in patients with AD compared with controls,[24,25] and because of its ease of use it should be investigated further as a screening test. These tests are summarised in Table 4.3.

Table 4.3   Clinical assessment and psychometric tests for detecting dementia

	Clinical diagnosis	CFFT	CRT
Low cost	-	+	+
Ease of use	-	+/-	+/-
Portable	+	+	+
Low risk	+	+	+
Detection of dementia	+	+	?
Detection of type of dementia	+	+/-	?
Established reliability	+	+	?
Useful in mild dementia	+/-	+	?
Useful in pre-clinical dementia	-	+/-	?

CFFT, Critical Flicker Fusion Threshold; CRT, Choice Reaction Time.

Electroencephalogram

The EEG is a potentially useful measure in patients with AD, and slowing of alpha frequency and increased theta and delta activity are observed as the condition progresses. Differences tend to be greater during rest with eyes open, and in one recent study the test was able to correctly classify 77% of patients with mild AD.[26]

Event-related potentials

Event-related potentials (ERPs) are changes in brain electrical activity, as recorded by scalp electrodes, in response to external stimulation of one of the many sensory tracts in the brain. Hence auditory ERPs can be recorded over the auditory brain cortex in response to the subject listening to an auditory stimulus. The subject is presented with two slightly different stimuli, one frequently and the other rarely (the 'oddball'). Signal averaging detects the potential generated in response to the 'oddball' (called the 'oddball ERP'). ERPs are plots of microvolts against time and have the appearance of several waves. Each component wave is named according to whether it is a negative (N) or positive (P) deflection. ERPs have been studied in a variety of conditions.

In a case–control study,[27] abnormalities in the 'oddball ERP' have been observed in those at increased risk for developing AD (i.e. those who have a family history of AD or who carry the apolipoprotein E ε4 allele) (see Chapter 3). These changes were observed in the absence of neuropsychological deficits. It therefore seems that AD has a pre-clinical stage and early detection should theoretically be possible. There is some evidence that in familial AD, episodic memory problems predate the onset of AD with clear signs of progression.[28] In this study, AD was diagnosed according to National Institute of Neurological and Communicative Disorders and Stroke, AD and Related Disorders Association criteria. This study showed that more subtle cognitive changes predate other more obvious cognitive changes. Some of the neuroimaging and electrophysiological techniques are summarised in Table 4.4.

Table 4.4 Neuroimaging and electrophysiological tests for detecting dementia

	MRI	CT	MRS	PET	EEG	ERP
Low cost	-	-	-	-	-	-
Ease of use	-	-	-	-	-	-
Portable	-	-	-	-	-	-
Low risk	+/−	+/−	+/−	+/−	+	+
Detection of dementia	+	+	+	+	+/−	+
Detection of type of dementia	+	+	+	+	+/−	+/−
Established reliability	+	+	+	+	+	+
Useful in mild dementia	+	+	+/−	+/−	+/−	+/−
	research centres	research centres	research centres	research centres	research centres	research centres
Useful in pre-clinical dementia	+/-	-	?	?	?	?

MRI, magnetic resonance imaging; CT, computerised tomography; MRS, magnetic resonance spectroscopy; PET, positron emission tomography; EEG, electroencephalogram; ERP, Event-related potential.

Biochemical tests

Acetylcholine, a neurotransmitter involved in memory mechanisms, is found predominantly in the cerebral cortex, caudate nucleus and parts of the limbic system. The presence of this neurotransmitter can be indirectly assessed by the presence of either the synthetic enzyme, choline acetyltransferase (CAT), or the metabolic enzyme, acetylcholinesterase (AChE). By measuring these enzymes, it has been shown that there is an age-dependent reduction in CAT and that CAT concentrations are also decreased in patients with AD, but these findings have not led to any clinically useful test.

A reliable serum marker for early AD and other causes of dementia would be helpful and a number of candidate markers have been suggested. Levels of α1-antichymotrypsin (a protein which is released from the liver during acute inflammatory states) have been measured in the serum and cerebrospinal fluid (CSF) of patients with AD and vascular dementia.[29] However, the study was relatively small, involving only 74 subjects. There was much overlap in the raised CSF levels between the three groups (AD patients, vascular dementia patients and the control group). However, raised levels above 0.75% of the total CSF protein were highly specific for AD, with a specificity of 100% but a sensitivity of only 25.6%. Larger studies would be useful to confirm this finding.

Tau protein and beta-amyloid in the CSF have also been suggested as possible markers for the early detection of AD and Blennow *et al.*[30] concluded that they are particularly useful for discriminating between age-associated memory impairment, depression and secondary causes of dementia. However, this is not a universal view and Green[31] has suggested that these markers do not have sufficient sensitivity and specificity for clinical use.

Another possibility is the AD-associated neuronal thread protein gene which encodes a 41 kD membrane-spanning phosphoprotein. This gene is overexpressed in AD and this is said to begin early in the course of the disease. This protein is released or secreted by dying cells into the CSF. These elevated levels can be detected and the most recent assay, termed 7cGold, has greater than 90% specificity and sensitivity.[32]

However, even if a CSF-based test proved to be helpful as a diagnostic test, this is unlikely to be helpful from a practical perspective for screening large numbers of people with mild or pre-clinical AD. It is time-consuming and relatively expensive. The procedure is invasive and uncomfortable, occasionally painful and potentially dangerous. At this stage this is unlikely to move beyond a potential research tool.

There has also been a long-standing interest in free radicals. These are atoms or molecules with one or more unpaired electrons and are particularly likely to arise in chemical reactions involving oxygen. When oxygen is chemically reduced, free radicals may be formed, including the superoxide and hydroxyl radicals. These interact with other molecules, producing new free radicals, and thus set in motion a 'chain reaction'. Such substances are particularly toxic to biological molecules (e.g. DNA and proteins) and, to deal with them, the body uses a number of natural defences including enzymes (e.g. superoxide dismutase) and antioxidants (e.g. vitamin E).[33] It has been suggested that free radical reactions are the cause of ageing and AD. This is said to be due to the progressive accumulation of irreversible damage caused by free radicals, but to date no clinically useful test has been developed. These are summarised in Table 4.5.

Brain biopsy

This is unlikely to ever be a viable screening test. It is an invasive technique and would raise a number of practical and ethical concerns, including patient safety, issues to do with the handling and storage of tissue samples, difficulties related to consent and problems associated with using the procedure on large numbers

Table 4.5 Biochemical, olfactory and biopsy tests for the detection of dementia

	Blood tests	CSF tests	Brain biopsy	Olfactory tests
Low cost	+/-	-	-	+
Ease of use	+/-	-	-	+/-
Portable	+/-	-	-	+
Low risk	+/-	-	-	+
Detection of dementia	-	+/-	+/-	+/-
Detection of type of dementia	-	+/- *	+	+/-
Established reliability	+	+	+	?
Useful in mild dementia	-	+/-	+/-	?
Useful in pre-clinical dementia	-	-	-	?

*The only established test is measurement of the protein 14-3-3 in CSF for Creutzfeld–Jacob disease.

of people. Although the microscopic examination of such samples is often portrayed as a diagnostic 'gold standard', it is frequently difficult to distinguish between brain changes seen in healthy older people and the pathological features of early AD. Some of the changes seen in healthy older people include decreased brain weight, decreased brain volume, dendritic loss, widening of sulci and ventricles, neuritic plaques, neurofibrillary tangles, and deposits of lipofuscin, aluminium, copper, iron and melanin. These changes are also the primary neuro-pathological features seen in AD.

During the first 50 years in healthy older people, grey matter is lost at a greater rate than white matter, but during the second 50 years, white matter is lost at a greater rate. The loss in patients with AD is similar but greater, i.e. there is a quantitative rather than a qualitative difference, and for these reasons some authors have suggested that AD may simply be an exaggeration of the healthy ageing process.

Neuritic plaques, the neuropathological hallmark of AD, are extracellular aggregates, 50–200 μm in diameter, within the neuropil of the brain (that part of the grey matter between neurones consisting mainly of neuronal processes). The main constituent of amyloid is amyloid β protein, which is also known as βA4 and Aβ. Hardy and Higgins[34] put forward the 'amyloid cascade hypothesis', in which they proposed that βA4 is directly or indirectly neurotoxic and that this leads to the development of neuritic plaques and neurofibrillary tangles, with subsequent neuronal cell death. βA4 is derived from another larger protein, called amyloid precursor protein (APP), which has several different isoforms and is a transmembrane protein. However, the exact function of APP is unknown, although it may be important in maintaining the integrity of synapses. Interestingly, it has been known for some time that patients with Down's syndrome (trisomy 21) who live into their fifties also develop neuropathological features of AD, and the gene for APP has been localised on chromosome 21. Neurofibrillary tangles are lesions within the cytoplasm of the perikaryon of medium and large pyramidal cells of the neo- and paleocortex. They occur less frequently in the subcortical nuclei. Under the electron microscope they can be seen as paired helical filaments, but precisely how they impair cortical function is not known.

Although the pathological features of AD are well known, it is unlikely that brain biopsy will be widely used because of practical and safety considerations, but also because of the considerable overlap with the changes seen in healthy ageing.

Olfactory tests

Deficits in both odour detection and odour identification occur in patients with AD.[35] Odour identification deficits arise earlier than odour detection problems, presumably because the latter requires less cognitive functioning than the former. The utility of olfactory testing for differential diagnosis of dementia is limited. However, against healthy controls, odour identification tests have a correct classification rate (sensitivity) of 83–100%.[36] Perhaps such tests, which only take 5–10 minutes to administer, should be seriously considered for use as part of the diagnostic work-up in AD and should be investigated more fully.

The usefulness of olfactory mucosal biopsy has been proposed for the early diagnosis of AD. However, there is controversy as to the usefulness of such a biopsy, since no pathognomic changes have been found to date.[37]

Olfactory detection decreases with increasing age, but this is significantly greater in patients with AD.[38]

Genetic tests

This is a rapidly developing area and will undoubtedly be important for increasing our understanding of the aetiology of AD. It is less helpful in terms of diagnosis as a positive test does not predict when an individual patient will develop the condition. However, if an increased risk is identified, patients could be carefully monitored, perhaps every six months, and treatment started as soon as symptoms develop. It could also be useful in pre-clinical treatment using an enriched sample. Such treatment would be unsuitable for the general population but reserved for those at high risk based on their genetic profile. In the near future it is also likely to become increasingly important in the field of pharmacogenetics, where a particular genetic profile might guide which drug is prescribed. For more information on the genetics of AD, see Chapter 3.

Conclusions

Early diagnosis of dementia is important for a number of reasons. There is considerable overlap between diagnostic and screening tests. Pencil and paper tests such as the MMSE should be used for screening and tests such as CFFT may have an additional advantage in very early detection. Other measures such as neuroimaging and biochemical tests are more suited to clarifying diagnosis after screening or for research.

Key points

- Early diagnosis of dementia is important to help patients and their families plan for the future and increase the chances that treatments will be effective.
- If detected early, some dementias can be reversed such as normal pressure hydrocephalus, some can be stabilised thus preventing further progression including vascular dementia, and some can have their progression slowed such as Alzheimer's disease.
- Simple screening tests that identify cognitive impairment combined with further investigations is currently the best strategy for diagnosing dementia and the different subtypes.
- There is currently no diagnostic test for Alzheimer's disease although a wide range of tests are currently being investigated.

References

1 Stewart R (1998) Cardiovascular factors in Alzheimer's disease. *Journal of Neurology, Neurosurgery and Psychiatry.* **65**: 143–7.

2 Bullock R (2002) New drugs for Alzheimer's disease and other dementias. *British Journal of Psychiatry.* **180**: 131–9.

3 Greenhalgh T (1997) *How to Read a Paper: the basics of evidence-based medicine.* BMJ Publishing, London.

4 Hsu YY, Du AT, Wiener MW *et al.* (2001) Magnetic resonance imaging and magnetic resonance spectroscopy in dementias. *Journal of Geriatric Psychiatry and Neurology.* **14**(3): 145–66.

5 Chetelat G and Baron JC (2003) Early diagnosis of Alzheimer's disease: contribution of structural imaging. *Neuroimage.* **18**(2): 525–41.

6 Frisoni GB, Rossi R and Beltramello A (2002) The radial width of the temporal horn in mild cognitive impairment. *Neuroimage.* **12**(4): 351–4.

7 Herol K, Salmon E, Perani D *et al.* (2002) Discrimination between Alzheimer dementia and controls by automated analysis of multicenter FDG PET. *Neuroimage.* **17**(1): 302–16.

8 Cagnin A, Brooks DJ, Kennedy AM *et al.* (2001) *In vivo* measurement of activated microglia in dementia. *Lancet.* **358**: 766.

9 Villareal DT and Morris JC (1999) The diagnosis of Alzheimer's disease. *Journal of Alzheimer's Disease.* **1**: 249–63.

10 American Psychiatric Association (1994) *Diagnostic and Statistical Manual of Mental Disorders* (4e). APA, Washington, DC.

11 World Health Organization (1992) *The ICD-10 Classification of Mental and Behavioural Disorders: clinical descriptions and diagnostic guidelines.* WHO, Geneva.

12 Folstein MF, Folstein SE and McHugh PR (1975) 'Mini Mental State': a practical method for grading the cognitive state of patients for the clinician. *Journal of Psychiatric Research*. **12**: 189–98.

13 Shulman KI (2000) Clock drawing: is it the ideal cognitive screening test? *International Journal of Geriatric Psychiatry*. **15**: 548–61.

14 Brooke P and Bullock R (1999) Validation of a 6-item cognitive impairment test with a view to primary care usage. *International Journal of Geriatric Psychiatry*. **14**: 936–40.

15 Mundt JC, Freed DM and Greist JH (2000) Lay person-based screening for early detection of Alzheimer's disease: development and validation of an instrument. *Journal of Gerontology: Psychological Sciences*. **55(B)**(3): 163–70.

16 Schmand B, Walstra G, Lindeboom J *et al.* (2000) Early detection of Alzheimer's disease using the Cambridge Cognitive Examination (CAMCOG). *Psychological Medicine*. **30**: 619–27.

17 Fowler KS, Saling MM, Conway EL *et al.* (2002) Paired associate performance in the early detection of DAT. *Journal of International Neuropsychology and Sociology*. **8**: 58–71.

18 Semenza C, Borgo F, Mondini S *et al.* (2000) Proper names in the early stages of Alzheimer's disease. *Brain Cognition*. **43**: 384–7.

19 Teng EL and Chui HC (1987) The modified Mini-Mental State (3MS) examination. *Journal of Clinical Psychiatry*. **48**: 314–18.

20 Mathuranath PD, Nestor PJ, Berrios GE *et al.* (2000) A brief cognitive test battery to differentiate Alzheimer's disease and frontotemporal dementia. *Neurology*. **55**: 1613–20.

21 Curran S and Wattis JPW (2000) Critical flicker fusion threshold: a potentially useful measure for the early detection of Alzheimer's disease. *Human Psychopharmacology*. **15**: 103–12.

22 Hindmarch I and Wattis JP (1988) Measuring the effects of psychotropic drugs. In: JP Wattis and I Hindmarch (eds) *Psychological Assessment of the Elderly*. Churchill Livingstone, Edinburgh, pp. 180–97.

23 Sherwood N (1994) *Effects of Nicotine on Human Psychomotor Performance*. PhD thesis, University of Leeds.

24 Simpson PM, Surmon DJ, Wesnes KA *et al.* (1991) The cognitive Drug Research Computerised Assessment System for demented patients: a validation study. *International Journal of Geriatric Psychiatry*. **6**: 95–102.

25 Miller E and Morris R (1993) *The Psychology of Dementia*. John Wiley & Sons, Chichester.

26 Stevens A, Kircher T, Nickola M *et al.* (2001) Dynamic regulation of EEG power and coherence is lost early and globally in probable DAT. *European Archives of Psychiatry and Clinical Neuroscience*. **251**: 199–204.

27 Green J and Levey AI (1999) Event-related potential changes in groups at increased risk for Alzheimer's disease. *Archives of Neurology*. **56**(11): 1398–403.

28 Fox NC, Warrington EK, Seiffer AL *et al.* (1998) Presymptomatic cognitive deficits in individuals at risk of familial Alzheimer's disease. *Brain*. **121**: 1631–9.

29 Licastro F, Parnetti L, Morini MC *et al.* (1995) Acute-phase reactant α1-antichymotrypsin is increased in cerebrospinal fluid and serum of patients with

probable Alzheimer's disease. *Alzheimer Disease and Associated Disorders*. **9**(2): 112–18.

30 Blennow K, Vanmechelen E and Hampel H (2001) CSF total tau, Abeta42 and phosphorylated tau protein as biomarkers for Alzheimer's disease. *Molecular Neurobiology*. **24**: 87–97.

31 Green A (2002) Biochemical investigations in patients with dementia. *Annals of Clinical Biochemistry*. **39**: 211–20.

32 de la Monte SM and Wands JR (2002) The AD7c-ntp neuronal thread protein biomarker for detecting Alzheimer's disease. *Front Bioscience*. **7**: 989–96.

33 Jorm AF (1990) *The Epidemiology of Alzheimer's Disease and Related Disorders*, pp. 54–76, 77–86, 151–70. Chapman and Hall, London.

34 Hardy JA and Higgins GA (1992) Alzheimer's disease: the amyloid cascade hypothesis. *Science*. **256**: 184–5.

35 Serby M, Larson P and Kalkstein D (1991) The nature and course of olfactory deficits in Alzheimer's disease. *American Journal of Psychiatry*. **148**: 357–60.

36 Morgan CD, Nordin S and Murphy C (1995) Odour identification is an early marker for Alzheimer's disease: impact of lexical functioning and detection sensitivity. *Journal of Clinical and Experimental Neuropsychology*. **17**(5): 793–803.

37 Kishikawa M, Sakae MIM, Kawaguchi S *et al.* (1994) Early diagnosis of Alzheimers? *Nature*. **369**: 365–6.

38 Lange R, Donathan CL and Hughes LF (2002) Assessing olfactory abilities with the University of Pennsylvania smell identification test: a Rasch scaling approach. *Journal of Alzheimer's Disease*. **4**: 77–91.

5

The role of the consultant in modern dementia services

Roger Bullock

Introduction

The modern old age psychiatry service is starting to look very different than the model that was created by the pioneers of the speciality; and thus the focus of the consultant within it will necessarily change as well. Old age psychiatry has moved from its humble origins in the back wards of the asylums to become a huge field with areas ranging from complex psychopharmacology through community outreach services in to palliative care.

In terms of creating a consultant base in the UK, old age psychiatry has performed well. Many psychiatry trainees are moving in to the field, especially those interested in the general medical overlap. The advances in the scientific knowledge around dementia and the introduction of new treatments have made the subject attractive and increasingly proactive. Further, the insistence by the Faculty of Old Age Psychiatry at the Royal College of Psychiatrists to provide sensible catchment area sizes has seen most new jobs having manageable numbers.

However, the eclectic nature of the work means that the demands on one individual to be a specialist and deliver all aspects of the job have expanded the consultant role dramatically. Many individuals now perform aspects of most branches of psychiatry, including:

- acute assessment and clinical diagnosis

- continuing assessment and long-term care

- rehabilitation

- community care

- assertive outreach

- crisis intervention

- memory clinic and cognitive assessment

- liaison work

- palliative care

- forensic assessments

- nursing home care

all of which are an individual specialism (often with a dedicated consultant in other areas of psychiatry and medicine), plus:

- Mental Health Act work

- understanding and implementing new and complex psychopharmacology

- reviewing, reflecting and changing practice.

On top of this comes education, audit, management and personal development time. So clearly now something must give, and sensible job plans need to be devised to maximise the potential of both the individual and the department. It would seem then that some form of sub-specialisation is becoming inevitable. This may not necessarily mean having whole jobs created to match the sub-specialised area, but to offer a balanced service the local areas need to agree special interests for the senior clinicians so that all the important parts of the field are covered appropriately.

When it comes to dementia, it is problematic that there is still no such thing as a dementia service. People with dementia may see a psychiatrist, geriatrician or neurologist, and often more than one depending on how they present or who is the most interested. In the UK, the old age psychiatrist can offer a comprehensive service, whereas the other specialities are more hospital based. But the dementia work in psychiatry is part of a larger service, and is addressed with variable emphasis depending on local resource and interest. This continues to happen even though Alzheimer's disease is the third commonest cause of death in the western world, and costs £5 billion plus per annum in the UK, with informal care costs estimated at double that.[1] To meet demand, dedicated consultants to manage dementia may soon become a feature in the health service – and can be drawn from any of the above specialities, provided they can work in a complex multidisciplinary system.

The need for such dedicated services is increasing and the logical solution is to create cross-organisational arrangements that make roles clear and avoid duplication. Getting involved strategically in the formation and running of a 'dementia action team'[2] will eventually become a primary role for any consultant involved in the treatment of dementia.

There are still problems in creating services where the consultant can be at their most effective. The drive for lower catchment areas has sometimes been at the expense of creating other community services. When this happens, although there may be the requisite number of consultants, they end up doing work that could be done by others, and the medical model is perpetuated. The whole nature of old age psychiatry is the multidisciplinary nature of its assessment and care. Within a multidisciplinary team, the doctor's main role is to provide diagnosis and treatment and contribute to the risk assessment. Other aspects of the patient's needs are often better assessed by other nursing, social work and therapy staff. Granted, the consultant's role is often to co-ordinate and in many cases to lead such teams, but that does not mean having to do most of the work themselves.

A second arising difficulty is really whom the dementia consultant now will view as their main peer group. Traditionally, old age psychiatry is part of mental health services. Clearly now, the speciality has ever closer links with geriatric medicine, especially in the UK with their grouping together in the National Service Framework (NSF) for Older People. Dementia is not really a psychiatric illness, it is a group of medical conditions that often have psychiatric sequelae. Alzheimer's disease has been traditionally boxed as a mental health problem, while Parkinson's disease is always considered medical. But the occurrence of psychiatric symptoms in both conditions is not that dissimilar, and the cognitive loss shares similar pathology. We must therefore start to consider where the old age psychiatry consultants are best placed, especially those who will work mainly with dementia. Remaining separated from geriatric specialists does not make sense, which means that a structural shift from mental health services may be inevitable. Though uncomfortable, this may be appropriate on several levels:

- Working-age mental health services have their own NSF and development agenda, which although is funded still seems to include the need to meet savings targets across all services, including old age, who get nothing in return.

- The acute hospital agenda means investment in programmes to help older people remain out of hospital. Many psychiatric services missed out on inter-mediate care money by not being closely involved enough with local geriatric services. Continuing opportunities exist in this area, if integrated planning can be achieved.

- The existence of the two types of geriatric services means that arguments about who does what, and more often who pays for what, become a barrier to good patient care.

- Old age psychiatry continues to absorb new work, especially with the advances in dementia treatment. This is not accompanied by any significant increase in funding (bar, perhaps, some cholinesterase inhibitor funding following the National Institute for Clinical Excellence [NICE] guidance).

Old age psychiatry is, in the main, integrating with social services. Both seem to be chronically underfunded and now the social service budgets may be charged for people who 'block' acute hospital beds, which will put at risk anybody at home who needs help, as the pot remains finite. Paradoxically, acute beds do not include the dementia assessment beds that often have delayed discharges as well. Integration with geriatric services may improve the whole system rather than create unhelpful sanctions in parts of it. It is a model that has worked well for child psychiatry in many instances, and has not affected their role within psychiatry or at the Royal College of Psychiatrists.

So the old age psychiatry consultant must now be looking at where they devote the bulk of their energy in terms of development and continuing professional development (CPD). If we create dedicated dementia expertise (full-time dementia consultants or at least defined dementia sessions), they must be part of a system that understands and meets the changing needs and demographics of this evolving patient group. To do this effectively and in a way that the commissioning authorities will understand, using an older people's service planning forum will be more productive than a mental health one. It is also probably true that for future CPD, a teaching session on stroke will prove more useful than one on borderline personality disorder. Clearly a balance is required, but at present mental health issues may be felt to predominate too much.

So the first tasks facing a dementia consultant will be to emphasise the dementia component of their work by asking:

- Can I help create dedicated dementia services across the area in which I have responsibilities to reduce duplication and increase service provision?

- Where should these services be based, and how should training, peer review and revalidation be worked in to them?

The clinical role of the dementia consultant

Relationships with other clinical services

The key resource a consultant has is their clinical training and skills, mixed with a degree of experience. Most old age psychiatrists have gone through a formal training scheme, which gives a general training in psychiatry and then specialisation as an old age psychiatrist. Many have also acquired other clinical experience, for example medical or general practice training. It is important to emphasise the specialist nature of the work, as mental health services at times do not include old age psychiatry as a specialist service in its own right and group it with general adult services. This leads to an impression that they are similar, with patients changing course as they get older.

This attitude is wrong on age, choice and ethical grounds. The best and simplest way to consider the difference between the services is that old age psychiatry is often associated with neurodegeneration, whereas general psychiatry is involved in neurodevelopmental issues. Thus, a case of depression presenting for the first time in a 60-year-old may be more likely to be due to cerebrovascular disease, which may in turn be a prodrome for vascular cognitive impairment. Such patients may show elements of pseudodementia. On the other hand, a fifth case of depression in a 70-year-old, who suffered their first episode at 30, will probably represent a further relapse in a chronic illness. The latter patient should have the choice to stay with services that they know, the former needs a different therapeutic evaluation (cardiovascular assessment and perhaps brain MRI), which an old age service is more likely to provide as the cognitive elements of the presentation will be investigated as well. Age should not be a factor – services must be based on need.

This is important when establishing the position of old age psychiatry in a mental health system, especially how dementia services will be delivered. Setting clear boundaries makes the role explicit, especially as most of the cases of dementia, of whatever age, are increasingly routinely seen by the old age department. Setting clinical boundaries is also important with the medical departments. The shortage of neurologists and increasing focus on rehabilitation by geriatricians means that they are more than happy for enthusiastic old age psychiatrists to get involved with and manage other patient groups, such as stroke, Parkinson's disease, Huntington's disease, multiple sclerosis and motor neurone disease. While this is the direction logically to get involved in, especially in the memory clinics, it must again be explicit and negotiated, otherwise core clinical time will be used up.

Clarity around what clinical work an individual can manage is important. In the past, the pride and belief that old age psychiatry treats this patient group better than anyone else, whether true or not, has led to an ever-increasing workload and expectations that are no longer deliverable. In order to maintain the position as key older people's champions, consultants need to define what they can and cannot do, otherwise resources will be consumed too quickly.

Proposed changes in the legal framework of assessing capacity may emphasise these points. If a formal framework is introduced, there may be an expectation that old age psychiatrists will perform all the assessments. This will be both impractical and impossible. This is a scenario where the consultant will need to train many others, from a variety of services, and only see those cases that are complex enough to require them. Anything less will mean the workload becoming impossible.

Memory clinics

The growth of memory clinics has helped clarify some of the overlap. In 1995, only 25 such clinics existed.[3] In 2000, this had grown to 120, reflecting mainly the introduction of drugs for dementia. Most of the memory clinics discussed in these surveys are found in old age psychiatry departments, with just a handful run by a geriatrician or neurologist.

However, the use of memory clinics is not without issue. They are potentially an expensive resource and represent a new service development in most areas. The clinics have had a strong focus on diagnostic procedures and pharmacological treatment, more so since NICE[4] allowed the introduction of cholinesterase inhibitors and provided some funding for drugs and infrastructure. This has led to earlier diagnosis, which in turn has brought the need for the development of new skills in the consultant. These include pre- and post-diagnostic psychological work, which is clearly needed as imparting information to the dementia sufferer is complex[5] and now breaking bad news to patients who can understand the diagnosis is a new part of the work. By bringing in a more holistic context, the clinics are losing their elitist research-based emphasis, and instead merging with the original psychosocial model of dementia care and becoming more mainstream. They may thus help to reduce a clearly perceived stigma, and make cognitive assessment more routine.

The doctor in the memory clinic may be drawn from psychiatry, geriatrics or neurology. It does not really matter which speciality, provided they are trained and aware of the medical issues in dementia assessment. These are not just diagnostic, but also centre on co-morbid conditions and the intricacies of treatment with the new anti-dementia drugs. In memory clinics, up to 90% of the dementia diagnoses will be made up of Alzheimer's disease or mixed dementia.[6] Vascular dementia and dementia with Lewy bodies are reported to be common in the population, but tend to present to the community team with predominantly non-memory symptoms. These dementias all have characteristic clinical histories and well worked out operational criteria to assist diagnosis.[7-9] This does still leave approximately 10% of other memory disorders to evaluate. While some have operational criteria, e.g. frontotemporal dementia,[10] others are important as they may have reversible elements which can be treated,[11] or factors which affect prognosis, e.g. malignancy.

The diagnosis of the type of dementia is clearly important, but so too is the differential diagnosis of dementia from other conditions. Early surveys suggest that a large number of attendees at a memory clinic are not suffering with dementia. In the UK the mean is 25%,[3] while in the US it is reported as 6%.[12,13] The commonest alternative diagnoses are worried-well, mild cognitive disorders and other psychiatric disorders, the main one being depression with prevalence rates found of 5–10%.[14,15] Depression has always been a confounder in memory work. Late-onset depression is associated with reduced cognitive scores in validated tests, while depression is concurrent in 20% of dementia cases.[16] It is also common in self-referring patients. Barker et al.[17] found this group had an average Geriatric Depression Scale score of 4.4 (borderline depression) with a consequent disproportionate concern about their memory problem.

The doctor also has some specific roles in the clinic. The knowledge of drugs and their side-effects, especially anticholinergic, is an important part of the initial assessment. Concomitant medication is an important part of the history. Many of the dementias involve reduced cholinergic function. Many drugs prescribed to the elderly for common medical conditions have anticholinergic activity. These include digoxin, warfarin, frusemide and prednisolone. Knowledge of these and using possible alternatives to reduce the anticholinergic load may contribute to both aiding the differential diagnosis and the management plan.

The psychiatric interview includes looking for depression and psychosis and the psychiatric phenomena that commonly occur.[18] Consequently the prescribing of antidepressants and antipsychotics in dementia for these symptoms requires skilful handling. The Mental State Examination is to evaluate the psychiatric state of the patient and elicit phenomenology that may help with the differential diagnosis. In early dementia, depression is a confounder that needs to be eliminated and/or treated. It is a common presenting feature in frontal lobe dementia, where it is found with apathy and withdrawal; and is frequent in the early stages of Alzheimer's disease. Thus detection is necessary as treatment may improve cognition. Psychotic features can occur in most dementias, with a frequency of up to

60%. Early fluctuating psychosis is a feature of dementia with Lewy bodies while delusions tend to occur in the mid-stages of Alzheimer's disease. Delusions are a frequent marker for presentation to the services and are associated with behavioural disturbance and predict future institutionalisation.[19] It is this complex mixture of psychiatric symptoms with the organic presentation that makes the old age psychiatrist such a key professional in these initial assessments.

Detailed medical examination, especially of the central nervous system, is a key component of eliciting co-morbid conditions and aiding differential diagnosis. The look of the patient gives important information, and neurological signs are definite clues. Signs of hypertension are important, e.g. in the fundi, as hypertension in mid-life is a risk for dementia, yet blood pressure may be normal in presenting patients. In people below 65, up to 20% of presenting patients may have a co-morbid condition that aggravates the underlying dementia and has a reversible cause, dropping to 5% once past 65. Many of these conditions, e.g. constipation and urinary tract infections, are increasingly common with age. Proper assessment is needed to screen for these, especially if sudden changes in condition occur.

Laboratory tests are required to evaluate the patient's state and look for reversible causes. It would be too expensive to routinely test for all conditions so expert clinical judgement should be the main indicator of what to use.[20] Larson et al.[21] showed that good judgement can offset 25–34% of costs. This is why the consultant is integral in the process.

Putting together a coherent and affordable memory clinic protocol is a key role of the consultant with co-ordinating responsibility. Memory clinics are attracting patients at an earlier stage of their illness, resulting in a need for more extensive investigation. This comes at a cost, over and above the time of the core staff. With no new money, this means that the overall pattern of traditional services may have to change. Consultants should now use their own sparse time in evaluating the early-presenting dementia patients, while allowing the community team to deal initially with the more nursing and socially biased needs of those unlucky enough to be referred too late on in the illness.

Finally, memory clinics have created a specialist service that is not found elsewhere in mental health services, and as such are recognised as new and different. They have targeted dementia, but many will assess the cognitive state of patients with schizophrenia, depression and Korsakoff's syndrome. This has emphasised the specialist nature of this type of work, with general psychiatry consultants asking for focused information on patients they are not now necessarily trying to hand over. This model has changed relationships with general psychiatrists, who now recognise that dementia consultants do have different skills. This has also started to alter the issue around graduate patients, as again assessments about suitability for transfer rather than straight transfer are becoming more usual.

Community dementia services

Patients presenting later in the illness still need many of the assessments detailed above, but extra information will now be gathered by performing some of the examination in the community setting. This has been the rationale for the community service models that are found throughout the UK, and the use of home visits is not disputed in the later-presenting patients with dementia. The patients are often not so well and making them travel to a hospital is often a hindrance to them and unnecessary. Consequently, the memory clinic should concentrate on patients above a defined cut-off, while below this the traditional home-based services continue. Again, agreed standardised assessments are easier to communicate, and much of the information at home can be gathered in advance of any necessary doctor's visit. With earlier treatment, hopefully this patient group will diminish in size, and the needs will change – reduction in this activity can be factored in to the business plans as a long-term release of resource.

The community mental health team (CMHT) is the fundamental part of the community services, and offers a variety of assessment and care options that should address most of the patients' and carers' needs, especially where health and social services have managed to integrate. Using the community team to assess the more advanced patients at home is highly appropriate for several reasons:

- Most of the patients' needs will be met by the non-medical specialities.

- The model provides the flexibility to meet the needs of those with dementia who live alone[22] and have different requirements.[23]

- Delay may be built in to a system that relies on a consultant visit as there is inevitably less of them than anyone else.

- The domiciliary system is expensive, and often used to get an appointment with the consultant for the least appropriate patients. When consultants syphon off these patients they compromise the relationship they have as part of the CMHT.

The dementia consultant needs to create a working system with the community team. Clearly, they will be one of the senior doctors of their own discipline and may lead it, either directly or through a broader role (e.g. clinical director). Again, a large component of this interaction may be arranging standardised assessments that everybody can use and understand. The Royal College of Psychiatrists recommends that a senior doctor is involved in every assessment of dementia. This may be impractical, especially if it is the first assessment, but will become more possible if time is saved by the relevant parts of the assessment being first performed by others that are just as qualified and able. Home visits therefore remain an essential part of the work, but as a planned part of the team activities, not as an isolated consultant event. Doctor-to-doctor referrals that bypass this process reduce the coherence of the team, and domiciliary visits undermine it, especially as many domiciliary requests are often for patients whose needs are subsequently found to be mainly non-medical.

Learner and educator

Working with trainees is an important part of the consultant's duties; but this is not a role to be taken on lightly as it involves more than having junior staff with varying degrees of responsibility and service commitment. To be involved in medical education needs an understanding of where the consultant sits in the learning model, and from this how they want to involve themselves in the trainee's education.

The consultant can view themselves as an expert at the top of their professional group, the resource for information in the field or the best-informed clinician. All may be true, but to remain so involves the self-realisation that continued learning is the key element in retaining specialist status. The McMaster University looked at how knowledge was assimilated in medical training up to consultant level and then underwent a gradual decline through the remaining working years. They felt that learning through enquiry and by means of medical epidemiology produced senior doctors who continued to learn rather than reproduce medical facts. Learning through enquiry does not stipulate limits, so the nearer to the edge of available knowledge one operates, the more specialist the knowledge retained. This learning technique generated evidence-based medicine. Much of this vogue is to be supported, but the insistence on having randomised, controlled evidence for everything is devaluing clinical experience and creating the notion that there is always a clear answer. This is not the case, and the extrapolation of what is known, in a sensible way, to the unknown is a specialist role that experiments with practice in a way that advances knowledge.

The advent of new treatments and changing patient demographics in dementia mean that education and learning are key responsibilities for the dementia consultant. With the constantly changing knowledge base, they must be active conveyors of these developments to the psychiatric trainees and the multidisciplinary staff. To be able to do so requires sensible job plans, which serve to encourage the individual and enhance the departmental good. The traditional totalitarian geographical job plan that is the basis of most new post needs updating to increase flexibility in the choice of component parts. If consultants can practise what they are interested in, they are more likely to perform well and utilise research and modern methodology. Trainees will benefit from this, and in turn can choose their clinical sessions from a menu of special interests rather than being aligned to just one consultant. This broadens their experience and makes them even more obviously supernumerary, as their alignment to just one team will be less. This allows the educational supervision to take place outside the straight hierarchy models, and should produce more rounded specialists at the completion of training.

The managerial role of the dementia consultant

The changing face of the services for dementia means that the consultant must be involved in all aspects of service change at managerial as well as clinical levels.

This input should be predominantly at strategic level, but consultants often end up as clinical directors/leads, where the responsibilities increase. Thus the managerial duties of a dementia consultant vary according to the managerial level they operate at:

- *Clinical director*: will be responsible for clinical governance in the department and may be involved with appraisals of both medical and non-medical staff. They may have budgetary responsibility and get involved in more operational matters. They are, in effect, the player/manager of the service. This is not necessarily a medical position.

- *Lead consultant*: will be the spokesperson of the medical group they work in. They will be responsible for collecting and conveying the general medical view, usually at strategic meetings with senior managers. The operational role will be limited and medically orientated – for example, looking at on-call rotas.

- *Consultant*: will need to represent their part of the service at local managerial meetings. They will need to ensure that the views of the staff they work with and their own ideas for the development of services are conveyed to the local management team, and report feedback in return. They are key players in ensuring the quality of local service provision and one of the principal advocates of good patient care.

What is clear is that consultants must engage in managerial issues. Financial pressure means that paper decisions are made that are sometimes not appropriate, and on occasion border on the unethical. To retain professional rigour, the consultant must be involved. Nothing gives a better example of this than the piecemeal introduction of cholinesterase inhibitors. Strong clinical involvement puts patients first and may offer alternative solutions through doing things differently rather than cutting pieces of service.

The NHS dementia consultant as a researcher

Research should not just be the province of the universities, and the NHS is trying to encourage more within mainstream work. New technology, drugs and models of care are continually being introduced now, and as a field the dementia specialists are keen to embrace them. If this is done in a systematic way then the data collected are useful and evaluable. Getting involved in larger projects should be encouraged too if time can be made, preferably by making research sessions part of some consultants' job plans.

Many aspects of dementia treatment have a reasonable evidence base, many more need good clinical research to ratify them. Memory clinics need audit and more research into the treatments that they offer. Clinicians should therefore measure what they do as practice continues to evolve. Local researchers should facilitate this as it keeps theory close to practice and ensures that patients get high-quality care, new research is properly implemented and new ideas arise. In short, any consultant who is regularly enquiring into their practice may make the next breakthrough to benefit an aspect of the care that those with dementia need.

Key points

- A great deal of the consultant's work in old age psychiatry is their involvement in caring for those with dementia. Single consultants with large catchments clearly cannot do it all and continue to develop effective services – trying to be clinician, educator, manager and researcher may be too much and the need to create achievable job plans based on the work needing to be done is ever more apparent.
- Consultants need to decide what they are best suited to do, what they can actually achieve and what is the best framework in which they can achieve it. Obviously, the balance of their selected job plan can change with time, and at the time new staff are added.
- The consultant role is changing, and will continue to do so, especially if the number of trainees available do not keep up with demand and other staff (e.g. nurses and psychologists) take on further responsibility. This chapter acts as a stimulus to consider how one's current job plan could be different. By using it to reflect on the current post and how it could be different, this is a resource for appraisals and planning of future posts.
- Ultimately we need dedicated dementia services. This will enable the consultant to have time to implement new models of care and new technologies as they become available. The management of dementia is going to be an ever-increasing field as the causes of cognitive decline become clearer and patients are treated earlier. Well-informed consultants with the capacity to deliver modern services will always remain central to what may prove to be some of medicine's most exciting developments.

References

1 Bosanquet N, May J and Johnson N (1998) *Alzheimer's Disease in the UK: burden of disease and future care*. Health Policy Review No. 12. Imperial College of Science and Technology, London.
2 Bullock RA (2002) *Building a Modern Dementia Service*. Altman, London.
3 Wright N and Lindesay J (1995) A survey of memory clinics in the British Isles. *International Journal of Geriatric Psychiatry*. **10**: 379–85.
4 NICE Technology Appraisal Guidance No. 19 (2001) *Guidance on the Use of Donepezil, Rivastigmine and Galantamine for the Treatment of Alzheimer's Disease*. Department of Health, London.
5 Drickamer MD and Lachs MS (1992) Should patients with Alzheimer's disease be told their diagnosis? *New England Journal of Medicine*. **326**: 947–51.
6 Zhu L, Fratiglioni L, Guo Z *et al*. (2000) Incidence of stroke in relation to

cognitive function and dementia in the Kungsholmen Project. *Neurology.* **54**(11): 2103-7.

7 McKhann G, Drachman D, Folstein M *et al.* (1994) Clinical diagnosis of Alzheimer's disease: report of the NINCDS-ADRDA Work Group under the auspices of the Department of Health and Human Services Task Force on Alzheimer's Disease. *Neurology.* **34**: 939–44.

8 Roman GC, Tatemichi TC, Erkinjuntti T *et al.* (1993) Vascular dementia: diagnostic criteria for research studies – report of the NINDS-AIREN international workshop. *Neurology.* **43**: 250–60.

9 McKeith I, Perry R, Fairbairn A *et al.* (1992) Operational criteria for senile dementia of Lewy body type. *Psychological Medicine.* **22**: 911–22.

10 Burn A, Neary O, Gustafson L *et al.* (1994) Clinical and neuropathological criteria for fronto-temporal dementia. *Journal of Neurology, Neurosurgery and Psychiatry.* **57**: 416–18.

11 Walstra GJ, Teunisse S, van Gool WA *et al.* (1997) Reversible dementia in elderly patients referred to a memory clinic. *Journal of Neurology.* **244**: 17–22.

12 Hogan DB, Theireer DE, Ebly EM *et al.* (1994) Progression and outcome of patients in a Canadian Dementia Clinic. *Canadian Journal of Neurological Sciences.* **21**: 331–8.

13 Weiner MF, Bruhn M, Svetlik D *et al.* (1991) Experiences with dementia in a dementia clinic. *Journal of Clinical Psychiatry.* **52**: 234–8.

14 Skerrit U, Pitt B, Armstrong S *et al.* (1996) Recruiting patients for drug trials: a difficult task. *Psychiatric Bulletin.* **20**: 708–10.

15 Ames D, Flicker L and Helme RD (1992) A memory clinic at a geriatric hospital: rationale, routine and results from the first 100 patients. *Medical Journal of Australia.* **156**: 618–22.

16 Ballard C, Bannister C, Solis M *et al.* (1996) The prevalence, associations and symptoms of depression amongst dementia sufferers. *Journal of Affective Disorders.* **36**: 135–44.

17 Barker A, Carter C and Jones R (1994) Memory performance, self-reported memory loss and depressive symptoms in attenders at a GP-referral and a self-referral memory clinic. *International Journal of Geriatric Psychiatry.* **9**: 305–11.

18 Burns A, Jacoby R and Levy R (1990) Psychiatric phenomena in Alzheimer's disease. *British Journal of Psychiatry.* **157**: 81–94.

19 Steele C, Rovner B, Chase GA *et al.* (1990) Psychiatric symptoms and nursing home placement of patients with Alzheimer's disease. *American Journal of Psychiatry.* **147**: 1049–51.

20 Terry RD, Katzman R and Bick KL (eds) (1994) *Alzheimer Disease.* Raven Press, New York.

21 Larson EB, Reifler BV, Sumi SM *et al.* (1986) Diagnostic tests in the evaluation of dementia: a prospective study of 200 elderly outpatients. *Archives of Internal Medicine.* **146**: 1917–22.

22 Social Services Inspectorate (1997) *Older People with Mental Health Problems Living Alone: anybody's priority?* SSI, London.

23 Alzheimer's Disease Society (1994) *Home Alone: living alone with dementia.* ADS, London.

6

The role of the clinical psychologist in the assessment, diagnosis and management of patients with dementia

Edgar Miller

Introduction

The very concept 'dementia' is psychological in that it implies, above all else, a deterioration in psychological functioning. It is this deterioration in mental functioning that is the central feature of dementia and results in the major practical problems posed by this group of disorders. For this reason, psychological factors are essential considerations in diagnosis and management for all those who deal with those who suffer from dementing illnesses. In this sense, the psychological aspects of dementia go much wider than the contribution made by psychologists, although there is clearly a role for the psychologist. It is the particular contribution of the clinical psychologist to the evaluation and management of those with dementia that is the focus of this chapter.

The practical contribution made by the psychologist has two major aspects. The first is that of the psychological assessment and diagnosis of dementia, often involving the use of psychometric tests. The second major contribution is to management. These two aspects will be considered separately.

Assessment and diagnosis

Psychological assessment of the person with dementia or possible dementia can be designed to achieve three possible aims:[1]

- as a means of assisting in the diagnosis of dementia
- to monitor change
- to make decisions about management.

Diagnostic assessment is the best developed of these areas and the present discussion will concentrate on this aspect and then make a few comments about other aspects of assessment.

Before commenting on assessments of different kinds, it is useful to draw attention to two sets of problems which complicate the psychological assessment of those with actual or possible Alzheimer's disease or other dementing illnesses.[2] Firstly, those assessed tend to be older and older people are subject to sensory loss and to physical problems, such as cardiovascular disease, which might impair psychological functioning.[3] Secondly, although the picture is improving, many potentially useful psychological tests do not have norms for older age groups and this presents a limitation on the range of instruments that can be used. This is especially a problem with regard to those who are over 75 or 80 years of age, although the situation is slowly improving.

Whilst these two problems apply generally, there is a further set of difficulties that emerges when trying to assess people from different language and cultural backgrounds. This is especially the case for those immigrants born outside the UK whose first language is not English, and for these there is, as yet, no satisfactory solution. Generally speaking, those members of immigrant communities who have been raised and educated in the UK tend to perform similarly on psychometric tests to the indigenous population, but they may still score a little less well on some instruments because of cultural differences.

Diagnostic assessment

A major underlying problem with diagnostic assessment is that diagnosis is a key issue at the point at which the individual first presents to services with problems, and this is usually early in the course of the disorder. At this time, any psychological changes are likely to be small, and a key difficulty is the problem of detecting small changes in psychological functioning, especially when it is typically the case that there is no reliable information as to how the individual might have performed on psychological tests prior to the onset of the possible dementing illness.

Screening tests

A number of screening tests for dementia have been developed. These tend to be administered more by psychiatrists than psychologists and they are mentioned for completeness. The best known of these and possibly the best validated is the Mini-Mental State Examination of Folstein et al.,[4] although there are a number of similar scales available. These tend to embody a series of questions incorporating such things as general knowledge questions (e.g. 'Who is the Prime Minister?') and very simple memory tasks. The MMSE emerges as having useful, if far from perfect, levels of validity,[5] and the key items in such scales which are most effective in discriminating those with dementia are questions relating to memory and orientation.

Intelligence

As already indicated, the term 'dementia' suggests a decline in psychological functioning and especially in intellectual or cognitive functions. This might suggest that intelligence tests would play a major role in the assessment of dementia. In practice, the role of intelligence (IQ) tests of the kind exemplified by the commonly used Wechsler intelligence scales is rather limited.[6] One important reason for this is technical, in that the methods used to construct intelligence scales mean that they are relatively insensitive in reflecting small changes in functioning. It is, of course, in the early stages of dementia, before deterioration has progressed very far, that diagnosis is most difficult and where the potential contribution that psychometric tests might make to diagnosis would be most useful. As dementia progresses, it becomes easier to diagnose on clinical grounds and the value of formal testing is reduced.

Another problem in the use of intelligence tests to detect dementia is that for most people being assessed there will be no accurate indication as to the pre-morbid level of intelligence, and without some indication of this it is difficult to say if any decline in IQ has occurred based on an assessment of current IQ. Various methods of determining pre-morbid IQ have been suggested but the most satisfactory so far has proved to be the National Adult Reading Test (NART). This was originally developed in 1978[7] but has been subsequently updated. Fuller discussions of the use of the NART to estimate pre-morbid intelligence are provided elsewhere.[8,9]

The NART works on the principle that the ability to read words appears to be highly resistant to deterioration, at least in the early stages of a progressive disorder like dementia. The test contains a set of 50 words whose spellings are irregular (e.g. 'naïve' or 'juggernaut') and which the person being tested would not be able to read out loud with correct pronunciation unless they were already familiar with the words. The ability to read irregular words in this way correlates highly with IQ and so performance on this test can be used to indicate pre-morbid IQ.

Memory

Commonly, the earliest change to be noted in someone who is developing dementia is in memory. The sufferer is noted to be more forgetful than used to be the case. In line with this, tests of memory have generally proved to be the most reliable early psychological indices of dementia. There are many different memory tests and again this discussion will be confined to a small number of examples with the works cited giving access to a much wider range of tests and a much more detailed analysis of their use in this context.

One of the most commonly used memory tests is the Wechsler Memory Scale which is now in its third major revision.[10] In brief, this consists of a number of subtests dealing with different aspects of memory (verbal vs. non-verbal, short-term vs. long-term, etc.). The fact that this is a commonly used scale means that published data on its use has become readily available and its coverage of different aspects of memory is more comprehensive than most alternative tests of memory. Its main disadvantage arises out of that comprehensiveness, in that the full scale does take a long time to administer, which might reduce its acceptability with elderly patients.

Other useful memory tests with some standardisation data for elderly people are the Recognition Memory Test[11] and the Rivermead Behavioural Memory Test.[12] The former is a recognition test where verbal stimuli (words) or non-verbal (faces) are presented and then have to be subsequently recognised. The latter is an attempt to develop a more 'ecologically valid' memory test that tries to mimic the memory demands of everyday life. For example, one subtest requires that the person tested remembers to carry out an action when cued to do so by a bell. Whilst the allegedly ecological relevance of the Rivermead test make it attractive, the levels of reliability of its subscales are less than would be desirable.

As indicated above, tests of memory have proved to be the most reliable of all psychological tests in detecting dementia and, therefore, any assessment of possible dementia needs to evaluate memory. However, two cautions should be noted. Firstly, for those who have always had low IQ levels (at around an IQ of 80 or below), poor performance on tests of memory can quite commonly occur in the absence of anything that might cause a memory loss. This makes memory testing for diagnostic purposes unreliable below this IQ level. Secondly, most of those who go to their doctors complaining of memory loss do not turn out to have dementia.[13] Usually they turn out to have some functional psychiatric disorder, commonly depression, or no disorder at all is ever identified. Interestingly, where a relative (often the spouse) complains of memory loss in the partner, this is rather more likely to be indicative of some form of dementia in the partner.

Other specific functions

Dementia produces deterioration in all psychological functions. In consequence, evaluation of almost any aspect of functioning can be of potential value in identifying dementia. Probably of most value in examining cases of potential dementia are tests of language and visuospatial ability.[14,15]

With respect to language, Miller set out the view that 'the first changes to be noticed are usually a general poverty of vocabulary and range of expression; speech becomes circumlocutory and repetitive ... dysphasic signs may also appear at some stage of the illness'.[16] Impairments in naming are common and can be readily assessed using such instruments as the Graded Naming Test.[17] The appreciation of spatial relationships similarly tends to decline and often from quite an early stage in the disease process. Benton has developed a useful instrument to assess visuospatial functioning.[18]

Test batteries and diagnostic systems

A number of more elaborate diagnostic systems for dementia have been developed and these rely on medical/psychiatric features as well as psychological measures. The two main British examples are the CAMDEX system[19] and AGECAT.[20] These take a considerable length of time to administer but offer high levels of diagnostic discrimination. They are often used as research tools.

Similar tools have been developed in America. One of the most prominent of these is provided by the NINCDS-ADRDA criteria.[21,22] These have similar advantages and disadvantages to the CAMDEX and AGECAT and are again most commonly used in research settings rather than routine clinical practice.

Whilst psychological assessment can make a valuable contribution to the identification or diagnosis of dementia, they, like other forms of assessment (clinical, radiological, etc.), are far from perfect for this purpose. In general terms, normal levels of performance on cognitive tests (of memory, language, etc.) can almost always be taken as excluding dementia (except for initially high-performing individuals in the very earliest stages). Poor performance on such tests has value in pointing to a dementing illness but should not be regarded as diagnostic on its own. This is because there are a number of other reasons why test performance can decline. For example, there is evidence that some people who are very depressed may do badly.[2]

A second caution is that psychological assessment on its own should not be regarded as a reliable indicator of the type of dementia. Whilst some studies have shown that, for example, multi-infarct dementia does give a different pattern of performance on psychological tests from that of Alzheimer's disease, the overlap between groups is considerable which makes the differentiation of individual cases difficult and subject to considerable error.

Finally, whilst it is the case that patients with different forms of dementia (e.g. Alzheimer-type as opposed to cerebrovascular) do tend to have slightly different patterns of performance on psychological tests, there is always considerable overlap between the different groups. This tends to make psychological assessment much more reliable as a means of identifying some form of dementing illness than it is in distinguishing the type of dementia should such be present.

Monitoring change

The measurement of ongoing change in dementia has potential importance both from the point of view of tracking change in the individual but also in the evaluation of possible pharmacological agents that may slow down or even halt the underlying pathological process. This presents considerable technical difficulties in terms of developing measures that will be sensitive to relatively small amounts of change in such functions as memory. These problems are discussed elsewhere.[1,23]

Planning management

Again this is something that cannot be described in detail due to limitations of space – a more detailed account is provided elsewhere.[1] Such things as scales to assess 'activities of daily living' as developed by occupational therapists and the general set of techniques known as 'behavioural assessment' can be utilised in making decisions about, for example, whether individuals can be relied on to do certain things for themselves or in determining whether special intervention programmes might be useful.[24,25]

Psychological interventions

Given that the causes of dementia lie in brain pathology, psychological interventions are not going to halt or reverse the underlying pathological processes. However, there is increasing evidence that psychological or psychosocial interventions can help maintain functioning in those who suffer from dementia, so allowing them to live as fully and independently as possible.

Environmental manipulations

The impact of the organisation and arrangement of residential units on the functioning of residents with dementia has been extensively demonstrated. For example, an early study showed that arranging the chairs in a ward dayroom so that they were grouped round small tables rather than set in lines, as had been the case, improved the level of social interaction between residents.[26]

More recent work has demonstrated the impact of enhanced stimulation.[27] This might be expected to be helpful in that many residential units provide little stimulation and an unchanging, monotonous environment. In one investigation, music appeared to be especially effective in increasing social interaction and enhancing the recall of personal information.[28]

As counter to the above, it has also been argued that overstimulation may be unhelpful for people with dementia and lead to confusion.[29] Many care settings can be rather noisy with too much going on around the person. The best practice would appear to involve the person in a level of activity that is appropriately stimulating and enjoyable without going to the extremes of monotony and understimulation, on the one hand, or a stimulus overload on the other.

Special forms of intervention

A number of special forms of intervention for people with dementia have been devised. The first and still possibly best known of these is reality orientation (RO).[27] In brief, this was based on the notion that a key problem in those with dementia is that they become disoriented for place, time and person. RO is then delivered in two ways. Firstly, 24-hour RO involves changes in the environment involving such things as use of notices and clear signposting of key locations around the ward. Staff in interaction with patients also stress information relating to orientation (e.g. by being assiduous in referring to an individual by name and mentioning the time when relevant). Secondly, there are special RO sessions in which small groups of residents meet with staff members on a regular basis for about 40 minutes at a time. Originally, these involved stressing information relating to orientation, i.e. starting by going round each member of the group by name, discussing things going on at the time of year (e.g. the presence of spring flowers) and so on. In some manifestations of RO, these activities have been greatly extended to include a wider range of things (e.g. what is happening in the world outside). Clearly the content of the sessions also needs to be adapted to the functional levels of the group members.

In general, it is the effect of RO sessions rather than 24-hour RO that has been evaluated.[27] There is good support for the notion that certain aspects of cognitive functioning are enhanced by RO sessions, and especially performance on tests of orientation. It is less clear that any more generalised improvements in cognitive abilities of more general functioning occur without any special training in the aspect of behaviour of concern.[30] Another limitation is that any gains for RO disappear once the sessions are withdrawn.

Other special techniques are reminiscence therapy and validation therapy.[27,31] The former is based on the notion that older people tend to reminisce, and there is a rationale for the use of memories from the past in that people with dementia can recall things from the distant past whereas they may not be able to remember what happened yesterday. Talking about the past in a group setting can then be used as a bridge to discuss issues relating to the present.

Validation therapy grew out of the belief of an American social worker (Naomi Feil) that RO and similar methods were too confrontational and led to the person withdrawing and possibly becoming hostile. This could well be at least as much a criticism of the routine and unthinking way in which interventions like RO have been applied in some settings as being necessary aspects of the techniques themselves. Validation therapy stresses the validation of feelings in whatever time or place appears to be real to the individual, regardless of whether this corresponds to what staff members regard as the 'here and now'. The widow who talks as if her husband is still alive may be responded to not by denying this but, for example, by pointing out that the listener is aware that she was very fond of her husband.

In terms of evaluation, reminiscence therapy is less well explored than RO, but the evidence of any kind of potentially beneficial outcome is not great. There do appear to be changes within sessions,[27] but these have not been shown to be manifest outside the sessions. Validation therapy has yet to be properly evaluated. Possibly its greatest benefit is to remind staff that apparently disordered utterances need to be handled sensitively.

This brief discussion does not exhaust the list of approaches that have been specially developed for use in dementia. Dementia care mapping[32] is one approach that has attracted much interest in the UK, although it so far has less to say as a specific approach to intervention as opposed to a way of assessment or evaluating quality of care. One key feature of all the approaches mentioned in this section as well as some others which have not been mentioned is worthy of comment. Although they can be varied to suit the needs of individuals, they are all based, implicitly or explicitly, on a particular assumption about the nature of a key problem in dementia (e.g. loss of orientation in the case of RO). A contrary point is that people with dementia do vary quite considerably and that what is the key problem (or set of problems) for one individual with dementia might not be the key problem(s) for another. In consequence, what are also required are methods of tackling problems relevant to individuals, and it is with such methods that the next section is concerned.

Interventions for individual problems

As already argued, people with dementia are different from one another and often have their own particular problems or difficulties, some of which may be amenable to psychological interventions. One class of such problems are those often referred to as 'challenging behaviour'.[33] Examples of challenging behaviour are aimless wandering, hoarding, refusing to bathe or wash, and so on.

Interventions to deal with such problems need to be specially designed on an individual basis in order to match the intervention to the nature of the problem, the characteristics of the individual concerned and the circumstances in which the problem arises. A wide range of potentially useful forms of intervention have been developed by clinical psychologists for use with other clinical groups, but which can be readily exploited and adapted to deal with the behavioural problems presented by those who suffer from dementia. These include such things as the behavioural and cognitive therapies.[25,34] However, these are best employed when the problem concerned has been subject to a careful functional analysis to determine the factors that enhance or reduce it.[35] Other means of ensuring that interventions match the needs of the individual involved such as analysing the problem graphically and evaluating the therapy process with the individual, have also been described.[36] There is evidence that such methods can be adapted successfully in work with those with dementia and that they can achieve at least some therapeutic goals.

General comment on interventions

The emphasis on developing psychological interventions for older people with dementia has been very much dominated by methods for use primarily in residential care settings, although there have been very occasional exceptions.[1] Given that a large proportion of those with dementia live in the community, often with some sort of support from relatives, more effort needs to be put into developing methods that can be used in the community. A useful model comes from the field of learning disability where a large literature has developed on ways of helping and training relatives (often parents) to develop simple strategies for themselves to deal with problems raised by severely learning-disabled family members.

Conclusions

This chapter has provided a brief outline of the contribution that psychological methods can make to the assessment and management of the person with dementia. Work in this area has become a rapidly expanding field. This chapter has set out to describe in outline some of the basic issues and space has precluded the detailed exploration of many aspects. This is especially so with regard to currently ongoing developments in the area of psychological interventions. The role of psychological assessment in dementia is much better established and this makes it easier to offer a reasonably definitive summary of this aspect.

Since dementia is biologically determined and progressive, it is clear that what can be achieved by psychological interventions alone is going to be limited. Nevertheless there is now good evidence that psychological or psychosocial interventions can at least help to maintain functioning and/or retard its decline. With recent and ongoing developments in the pharmacological treatment of dementia, the role of psychological interventions is likely to become enhanced. If pharmacological agents can slow down or even halt the underlying pathological process, this means that it is likely that those who suffer from dementia will tend to remain mildly impaired for much longer. Other forms of intervention, such as those of a psychological nature, that can help such people live as fully and independently as possible will then need to be used in tandem with pharmacological treatments if the overall quality of life of sufferers is to be maximised.

Key points

- Psychological assessment can make a useful contribution in the diagnosis of dementia, but like other methods for detecting dementia is not wholly accurate, and so evidence from psychological assessments needs to be considered in the context of other possible indicators.
- Within psychological forms of assessment, tests of memory offer the best single indicator of the presence of dementia.
- Psychological assessment is not very useful for discriminating between different forms of dementia.
- There is good evidence that even people with quite marked levels of dementia are sensitive to environmental influences. For example, even such simple things as the arrangement of furniture can have an effect on the amount of verbal interaction between residents in a residential unit.
- A number of specially designed forms of intervention for use with those suffering from dementia have been devised. The best known and best validated of these is reality orientation, but even here the gains are limited and short-lived after the programme has been discontinued.
- Special forms of intervention, such as reality orientation and reminiscence therapy, tend to assume that all those suffering from dementia share a single key disability or feature. This assumption may not be entirely true and the use of more specific forms of psychological intervention of the kinds used with other client groups should be considered in order to address the specific problems of individuals.

References

1 Miller E and Morris R (1993) *The Psychology of Dementia*. John Wiley & Sons, Chichester.

2 Miller E (1996) The assessment of dementia. In: RG Morris (ed.) *The Cognitive Neuropsychology of Alzheimer-type Dementia*. Oxford University Press, Oxford.

3 Hale WE, Stewart RE, Moore MT *et al.* (1992) Electrocardiographic changes and cognitive impairment in the elderly. *Journal of Experimental and Clinical Gerontology.* **14**: 91–102.

4 Folstein MF, Folstein SE and McHugh PR (1975) Mini-Mental State: a practical method for grading the cognitive state of the patient for the clinician. *Journal of Psychiatric Research.* **12**: 189–98.

5 Teng EL, Chui HC, Schneider LS *et al.* (1987) Alzheimer's dementia: performance on the Mini-Mental State Examination. *Journal of Consulting and Clinical Psychology.* **55**: 96–100.

6 Wechsler D (1997) *Wechsler Adult Intelligence Scale III*. Psychological Corporation, San Antonio, TX.

7 Nelson H and O'Connell A (1978) Dementia: the estimation of premorbid intelligence using the new adult reading test. *Cortex.* **14**: 234–44.

8 Crawford JR (1992) Current and premorbid intelligence measures in neuropsychological assessment. In: JR Crawford, DM Parker and WW McKinlay (eds) *A Handbook of Neuropsychological Assessment*. Lawrence Erlbaum, Hove.

9 Morris RG and Kopelman MD (1992) The neuropsychological assessment of dementia. In: JR Crawford, DM Parker and WW McKinlay (eds) *A Handbook of Neuropsychological Assessment*. Lawrence Erlbaum, Hove.

10 Wechsler D (1997) *Wechsler Memory Scale III*. Psychological Corporation, San Antonio, TX.

11 Warrington EK (1984) *Recognition Memory Test*. NFER-Nelson, Windsor.

12 Wilson B, Cockburn J and Baddeley AD (1985) *The Rivermead Behavioural Memory Test*. Thames Valley Test Co., Reading.

13 O'Brien JT, Beats B, Hill K *et al.* (1992) Do subjective memory complaints precede dementia? A three-year follow-up of patients with 'benign senescent forgetfulness'. *International Journal of Geriatric Psychiatry.* **7**: 481–6.

14 Coslett HB and Saffran EM (1996) Visuospatial functioning. In: RG Morris (ed.) *The Cognitive Neuropsychology of Alzheimer-type Dementia*. Oxford University Press, Oxford.

15 Emery VOB (1996) Language functioning. In: RG Morris (ed.) *The Cognitive Neuropsychology of Alzheimer-type Dementia*. Oxford University Press, Oxford.

16 Miller E (1989) Language impairment in Alzheimer-type dementia. *Clinical Psychology Review.* **9**: 181-95.

17 Warrington EK and McKenna P (1983) *Graded Naming Test*. NFER-Nelson, Windsor.

18 Benton AL, Varney NR and Hamsher K (1978) Visuospatial judgement: a clinical test. *Archives of Neurology.* **35**: 364–7.

19 Roth M, Tym E, Mountjoy CQ *et al.* (1986) CAMDEX: a standardised instrument for the diagnosis of mental disorder in the elderly with special refer-

ence to the early detection of dementia. *British Journal of Psychiatry*. **149**: 698–709.

20 Copeland JRM, Dewey ME and Griffith-Jones HM (1986) A computerised diagnostic system and case nomenclature for elderly subjects: GMS and AGECAT. *Psychological Medicine*. **16**: 89–99.

21 Blacker D, Albert MS, Bassett SS *et al*. (1994) Reliability and validity of NINCDS-ADRDA criteria for Alzheimer's disease. *Archives of Neurology*. **51**: 1198–204.

22 McKhann G, Drachman D, Folstein M *et al*. (1984) Clinical diagnosis of Alzheimer's disease: report of the NINCDS-ADRDA Work Group under the auspices of the Department of Health and Human Services Task Force on Alzheimer's Disease. *Neurology*. **34**: 939–44.

23 Miller E (1992) Some basic principles of neuropsychological assessment. In: JR Crawford, DM Parker and WW McKinlay (eds) *A Handbook of Neuropsychological Assessment*. Lawrence Erlbaum, Hove.

24 Kuriansky JB and Gurland BJ (1976) The performance test of activities of daily living. *International Journal of Aging and Human Development*. **7**: 343–52.

25 Kazdin AE (1975) *Behavior Modification in Applied Settings*. The Dorsey Press, Homewood.

26 Sommer R and Ross H (1958) Social interaction on a geriatric ward. *International Journal of Social Psychiatry*. **4**: 128–33.

27 Woods RT (1996) Psychological 'therapies' in dementia. In: RT Woods (ed.) *Handbook of the Clinical Psychology of Ageing*. John Wiley & Sons, Chichester.

28 Lord TR and Garner JE (1993) Effects of music on Alzheimer patients. *Perceptual and Motor Skills*. **76**: 451–5.

29 Cleary TA, Clamon C, Price M *et al*. (1988) A reduced stimulation unit: effects on patients with Alzheimer's disease and related disorders. *Gerontologist*. **28**: 511–14.

30 Hanley IG, McGuire RJ and Boyd WD (1996) Reality orientation and dementia: a controlled trial of two approaches. *British Journal of Psychiatry*. **138**: 10–14.

31 Woods RT (1996) Cognitive approaches to the management of dementia. In: RG Morris (ed.) *The Cognitive Neuropsychology of Alzheimer-type Dementia*. Oxford University Press, Oxford.

32 Kitwood T (1993) Towards a theory of dementia care: the interpersonal process. *Ageing and Society*. **13**: 51–67.

33 Stokes G (1996) Challenging behaviour in dementia: a psychological approach. In: RT Woods (ed.) *Handbook of the Clinical Psychology of Ageing*. John Wiley & Sons, Chichester.

34 Woods RT (2000) *Psychological Problems of Ageing: assessment, treatment and care*. John Wiley & Sons, Chichester.

35 Sturmey P (1996) *Functional Analysis in Clinical Psychology*. John Wiley & Sons, Chichester.

36 Petermann F and Muller JM (2001) *Clinical Psychology and Single-case Evidence: a practical approach to treatment planning and evaluation*. John Wiley & Sons, Chichester.

7

The role of the physician for the elderly in the assessment, diagnosis and treatment of patients with dementia

Michael A Carpenter

Introduction

Dementia is a heterogeneous group of diseases that places a heavy burden on health and social services and especially informal carers. Patients with dementia have often been seen as a lost cause because of the incurable nature of the disease. However, incurable does not mean untreatable. It is vital that patients with dementia are treated with proper respect to themselves as people and to their disease. Proper support and advice for sufferers and carers can often maintain the patient in their own environment.

We now have drug treatments that can ameliorate some of the symptoms for a proportion of sufferers, at least temporarily. There are also secondary prevention strategies that may delay the progression of some of the underlying diseases. Patients with the so-called reversible dementias are a third group of patients that will be specifically addressed.

All clinicians that manage patients with dementia should recognise the importance of a proper diagnosis, a proper management plan and attention to the small factors that may improve the quality of life of the patient and their carers.

Patients with dementia usually present to the physician in one of two ways: as a patient with cognitive impairment in need of a diagnosis, or as a patient referred with another condition for whom their dementia may cause significant problems with the management of that condition. Many patients with dementia present as acute medical admissions to hospital with a preliminary diagnosis of 'failure to cope', and are frequently mislabelled as social problems.

The two groups of patients represent differing challenges to the physician and the chapter will consider them separately. There is an overlap between the two groups, in the sense that patients with dementia admitted to hospital may not have had their dementia fully assessed prior to admission, so the group of patients referred for assessment/diagnosis will be considered first. A detailed discussion of the aetiology and diagnostic criteria for dementia is outside the scope of this chapter. However, one cannot discuss the management of these patients without reference to the different diagnostic features. Furthermore, the role of screening for reversible dementias will be discussed.

Reversible dementia syndromes

There are a number of illnesses that may be associated with a dementia-like picture. Some of these conditions are treatable, and this raises the question as to whether treatment of the underlying disease may produce an improvement in cognitive function. Where the answer is yes, a missed diagnosis may lead to an irreversible decline and represent a missed opportunity to prevent dementia. The possibility of missing such an opportunity has led to an inordinate emphasis amongst physicians on this group of dementias. However, this group is a very small proportion of the whole, and the cost-effectiveness of screening for the group is not clear.[1] There is the added complication that many of the conditions listed are also accepted causes of acute confusional states. It is possible that the improvement in cognitive function of patients treated for reversible dementia may in part be due to the treatment of an acute confusional element superimposed on an underlying dementia.

The diseases most commonly included in the group of reversible dementia are shown in the Box 7.1.

Box 7.1   Causes of reversible dementia

- Hypothyroidism
- Vitamin B_{12} deficiency
- Folate deficiency
- Neurosyphilis
- Normal pressure hydrocephalus
- Frontal meningioma
- Hyperparathyroidism

The diagnosis of myxoedema madness is old and predates any form of biochemical testing for hypothyroidism or curative therapeutic options. Some studies have shown a striking response rate to treatment of hypothyroidism,[2] thus highlighting the importance of making a positive diagnosis. However, a more recent review suggests that rigorous application of diagnostic criteria for hypothyroidism may reduce the frequency of the diagnosis,[3] and most studies report improvements rather than cures. Physicians for the elderly would still routinely check thyroid function of patients with an unexplained decline, particularly if it has not been done in the last 12 months, even though the evidence is poor. Signs and symptoms of thyroid disease in the elderly are often non-specific and testing thyroid function in older people without cognitive impairment often reveals unsuspected abnormalities. It may be that this is a case of two common illnesses occurring in the same person.

Recent studies on the cost-effectiveness of testing for vitamin B_{12} give conflicting results. The prevalence of low B_{12} on serological testing in elderly populations varies from 3–15%, though there is uncertainty as to the significance of this finding in the absence of signs of deficiency.[4] In a review of the literature, 86% of patients shown to have low B_{12} levels have either anaemia or a raised mean cell volume (MCV).[5] In essence, the evidence for screening all patients with dementia for B_{12} levels is poor, and it seems reasonable to save B_{12} estimation for those patients with any one of anaemia, raised MCV or neurological signs suggestive of possible B_{12} deficiency. These include delirium, reduced vibration sense in the legs (which is common in the elderly anyway) and gait abnormalities suggestive of a spastic paraparesis (together manifesting as subacute combined degeneration of the cord).

In the absence of megaloblastic changes there are also difficulties in confirming the diagnosis of B_{12} deficiency with certainty.[6] The measurement of serum B_{12} is currently by bioassay and cross-reactive substances have been postulated that may give falsely high readings. A patient with low normal results may, therefore, be B_{12} deficient. It has been suggested that additional assays of homocysteine and methylmalonic acid may be required in these circumstances to assess tissue response to B_{12} deficiency.[7]

The value of treatment is also unclear.[6] Better trials are needed, but it seems likely that those with a shorter duration of symptoms, especially less than six months, are more likely to benefit. In this group, complete responses have been seen. Those with symptoms for more than 12 months are unlikely to improve significantly. The duration of symptoms also seems to be important in how rapidly a response will be seen. The haematological abnormalities may take up to two months to return to normal, and at least this length of time should be allowed before accepting a lack of response to treatment.

The evidence for folate deficiency and reversible dementia is even less clear-cut. There are no clear trials, but there is anecdotal evidence that giving folate to patients with neurological signs and symptoms of B_{12} deficiency, but with normal B_{12} levels, may result in a striking improvement.[8] It is worth considering as a diagnostic test in those circumstances, and in those patients with a poor dietary intake, where folate deficiency may be secondary to their dementia.

There is a significant debate about routine serological testing for syphilis for patients with cognitive impairment.[9–11] Less than 5% of elderly patients have positive serological tests on admission to hospital. In a study of 592 consecutive medical and psychiatric admissions aged over 65, 23 were found to have positive serology.[9] A third of those had been treated previously, 20% died of another condition shortly after admission and 17% (four patients) were given a curative course of antibiotics. Treatment was deemed inappropriate in the remainder for a number of clinical reasons. Treatment of syphilis is indicated on the basis of clinical picture and serological tests. For a diagnosis of active neurosyphilis, this requires positive serology in the cerebrospinal fluid.[12] This may be difficult in frail patients, especially if they are likely to be restless during the procedure. Even after lumbar puncture, treatment may only be indicated if the clinical picture is suggestive of neurosyphilis. It is reasonable, therefore, that unless there is an indication to suggest a diagnosis of neurosyphilis, serological testing with Treponema Pallidum Haemaglutination (TPHA) is not cost-effective.

Normal pressure hydrocephalus is another difficult area. Patients present with a triad of signs and symptoms: gait apraxia, urinary incontinence and cognitive decline. CT brain scan shows a dilated ventricular system with no effacement of the sulci. Unfortunately, a similar pattern can be seen in small-vessel vascular disease causing periventricular ischaemia. Ischaemic changes in the latter are usually visible within the white matter, but care should be taken to differentiate the two conditions. There is no single diagnostic test, and since the treatment is surgical with a mixed outcome, a careful assessment is required before embarking on treatment.

Inserting a ventricular shunt for normal pressure hydrocephalus may be associated with improvement. This is more likely when the hydrocephalus is secondary to a previous intracranial event, or where the gait apraxia and urinary incontinence predominate. However, the procedure carries with it a significant risk of morbidity (e.g. shunt infections, blockage, shunt nephritis). Anecdotally, a 'rule of thirds' is accepted: about one-third improve, one-third are unchanged and one-third deteriorate. Therapeutic lumbar puncture has been advocated, but the procedure shows no correlation with outcome from surgical shunting. Where cognitive decline is the predominant symptom, the outcome is more likely to be unfavourable.

Hypercalcaemia may be associated with a number of neuropsychological disturbances, and the role of hyperparathyroidism in dementia has been questioned. Patients with significant hypercalcaemia may have a delirium responsive to lowering the serum calcium, but parathyroidectomy has not been shown to be beneficial for those patients with established dementia.

The diagnoses historically called reversible dementias are therefore a small group of conditions, for which treatment at best can be expected to improve rather than cure cognitive impairment. It is reasonable, therefore, to concentrate on better diagnosis and management of the common dementias, rather than diverting too much time and attention to the reversible dementias. It is worthwhile screening for thyroid disorders, and assaying serum B_{12} and red cell folate levels, when the patient has anaemia or macrocytosis on full blood count, or neurological signs. TPHA should only be requested when the history or clinical signs suggest infection is likely. Serum calcium level is unlikely to help in the diagnosis of dementia, but is worthwhile when the diagnosis of delirium is suspected.

Assessment and diagnosis

The physician for the elderly has an important role in making the diagnosis of a dementia syndrome. General practitioners are often faced with a dilemma of whether they should refer patients with cognitive impairment to a physician or a psychiatrist. This difficulty arises partly through the possibility of delirium as opposed to dementia. Delirium is clearly within the domain of the physician, whilst dementia is now usually within the realm of the memory clinic run by the psychiatrist. It is not uncommon for a physician to make a diagnosis of dementia in a patient referred with a non-specific decline, in which the cognitive problems have not been previously recognised.

Patients are often referred because of increasing forgetfulness. The patient's perception of forgetfulness is not as reliable as a carer's perception, so corroborative evidence is vital.[13] Evidence of cognitive impairment does not in itself diagnose dementia. A history of the onset, duration and progression of the forgetfulness, and any associated features, is needed. If the onset of symptoms is acute, or the course of the illness has been fluctuating, a history of changes in conscious level must be sought. If the patient is forgetful, these facts will usually require the help of a third party. Where patients are admitted acutely to hospital with confusion, there is often co-existent delirium and dementia.[14] Only after treating the delirium can the dementia be properly diagnosed and managed.

It is not uncommon to find that dementia is the underlying diagnosis for patients referred because of falls, decreasing mobility, difficulty coping or even weight loss. It is mandatory, therefore, to carry out an assessment of cognitive function as part of any assessment of an older patient presenting with non-specific symptoms.[5] Clearly, it is important to exclude other causes of these conditions even where it is clear that the patient has a previously undiagnosed dementia.

Other features that may be of interest include the presence of symptoms such as speech disorders or motor problems, dyspraxias or mood disorders. The presence of speech disorders, such as non-fluent dysphasia, dysarthria or echolalia, may suggest underlying cerebrovascular disease or a frontotemporal lobe syndrome, though the latter is more commonly associated with a younger onset. If a patient has a pill-rolling resting tremor and bradykinesia, this would suggest Parkinson's disease (PD). A history of myoclonic jerks and a rapid decline may suggest Creutzfeld–Jakob disease (CJD), which is usually the sporadic variety rather than the BSE-related variant CJD in this age group. The doctor should also ask about symptoms of thyroid disorders, particularly those of hypothyroidism, though the classical symptoms are often absent in older people.

When examining patients with suspected dementia, the physician should look for signs of anaemia, thyroid disease and focal neurological disease (see Case Study 7.1), in particular, the presence of a hypothyroid facies, bradycardia and slow relaxing reflexes, suggestive of hypothyroidism. Blood pressure measurement is required, especially if the patient's dementia turns out to have a vascular aetiology, as treatment of the blood pressure may delay further vascular insults and worsening cognitive status.

In the neurological system, attention should be paid to higher functions, particularly speech and ability to perform tasks on request. The physician should look for constructional dyspraxias by assessing skills such as clock drawing and copying shapes, and test the ability to carry out second and third-order commands to assess the patient's ability to sequence activities. The simplest test is to ask the patient to take a piece of paper, fold it and put it down. The physician should also look specifically for pyramidal signs to suggest anterior circulation stroke, or basal ganglia signs such as rigidity or poor postural stability, that may indicate lacunar strokes. PD should be considered if there is a pill-rolling

---

Case Study 7.1

An 88-year-old woman was admitted from home after a fall. Examination revealed significant cognitive impairment, with an Abbreviated Mental Test score (AMTS) of 3/10, but was otherwise unremarkable. Routine investigations revealed marked hypothyroidism, and she was commenced on replacement therapy immediately.

A history from her informal carer subsequently revealed increasing forgetfulness for many months, to the extent of leaving pans on the cooker to burn dry, or lighting the gas cooker and hanging wet towels over it to dry.

Over the following six weeks her thyroid function returned to normal and her cognitive function improved. Her AMTS only rose to 7/10, indicating persistent cognitive impairment. She remained incontinent of urine despite regular toileting and denied this was a problem. However, the patient still lacked the ability to carry out simple domestic tasks when assessed in her own home. She was unable to sequence simple tasks without frequent prompting, and was unaware of the risks she was taking, e.g. leaving the gas cooker unlit whilst trying to boil a kettle.

---

resting tremor, rigidity, bradykinesia or other features such as micrographia. However, it is unusual for dementia to develop before the physical symptoms in PD.

Investigations should include a search for common physical illnesses, including estimation of haemoglobin, erythrocyte sedimentation rate, urea and electrolytes, glucose, thyroid function, and if the patient is anaemic or macrocytic, vitamin B_{12}. Where there is a history to suggest the possibility of sexually transmitted diseases, or signs to support a diagnosis of syphilis, TPHA should also be checked. If the patient has hypertension or ischaemic heart disease an ECG should be carried out. Left ventricular hypertrophy indicates a higher risk of cerebrovascular disease.

All patients with suspected dementia should have a CT or MRI brain scan, though which will depend on local availability. The presence of diffuse ischaemic changes will suggest a vascular basis for the disease, although co-existent Alzheimer's disease cannot be excluded. The presence of excessive global cerebral atrophy, although not diagnostic would, in a patient with a history of progressive cognitive impairment and in the absence of another cause, support a diagnosis of Alzheimer's disease. The presence of localised atrophy in the frontal and temporal lobes suggests a fronto-temporal dementia. Imaging will occasionally reveal an unsuspected space-occupying lesion.

Where the primary diagnosis is unclear, for instance where CJD, fronto-temporal dementia or other condition is suspected, referral to a neurologist for further diagnosis should be considered. Suspected CJD requires an EEG and lumbar puncture, with a sample sent to the CJD surveillance centre in Edinburgh for analysis.

The physician has a duty to discuss the diagnosis with the patient and carers. The patient should be given appropriate information on what may happen in the future and what can be done to try and ameliorate the symptoms and perhaps slow the disease. Time should be set aside for the purpose, with a suitable adult also present, usually the patient's next of kin or main carer. In light of the different treatments and secondary prevention strategies available, giving patients the specific diagnosis is now a prerequisite of good care.

Many physicians will commence treatment, while in other areas referral to a specific memory clinic may be more appropriate. This will often depend on local provision. If the physician plans treatment, then they must also ensure appropriate support for patient and family, either through community psychiatric nursing services or voluntary agencies such as the Alzheimer's Society. The physician must also regularly review the effectiveness of whatever treatment is commenced.

The regular assessments required by NICE guidance for patients with Alzheimer's disease given anti-dementia drugs often means that a formal service is required, and rather than attempt to reproduce this model, many clinicians will refer patients with this diagnosis to a memory clinic.

For other diagnoses the physician will often institute the medical treatment. Treatment of vascular dementia is primarily aimed at secondary prevention. Patients should stop smoking and blood pressure should be assiduously controlled, as should diabetes mellitus. Although there is no clear evidence that aspirin delays the progression of dementia associated with small-vessel cerebral ischaemia,[15] it is reasonable to extrapolate from the evidence for large-vessel disease and treat with aspirin 75 mg daily. Evidence has recently been presented that the combination of perindopril and indapamide may reduce the development of dementia in patients who have previously suffered a stroke.[16] The main aim of the trial was to show that treatment with these agents reduces the incidence of recurrent stroke. The effect on development of dementia was a secondary end-point and only reached significance in those who suffered a further vascular event whilst in the trial. The implication is that the combination of perindopril and indapamide reduces the risk of recurrent stroke, but for those patients who do suffer further vascular events, the risk of developing dementia is reduced.

Dementia and acute admission to a general hospital

Dementia is common amongst older patients admitted to hospital.[14] With as many as a third of all older patients suffering from delirium or dementia, assessment of the mental state of all patients is essential. The simplest assessment tool validated in the hospital setting is Hodkinson's abbreviated mental test.[17]

Patients with dementia in hospital provide a number of challenges, and staff should be aware of their needs. In the UK, the National Service Framework for Older People requires that patients with mental health problems in acute general hospitals are cared for by staff with appropriate training.[18] Patients with dementia have the right to be treated with the same respect as all other patients. Very often the patient may exhibit a stereotypical behavioural trait, such as echolalia or perseveration of speech. Healthcare workers should restrain the impulse to caricature such patients or encourage regressive behaviour.

Many patients with dementia become acutely confused and disoriented, either directly due to the pathology leading to admission or due to the change of environment. The noisy hospital environment, with the constant movement of personnel and frequent ward moves, is probably the worst way to manage a confused patient. Wherever possible, patients should be managed in a quiet area, with only familiar visitors in the early stages. Once the patient's trust has been gained, more people can have contact with the patient and exposure to the general environment can be gradually increased.

The physician should resist the temptation to sedate or restrain the patient. Very often these policies will have a detrimental effect. Over-sedation will render the patient unable to care for themselves, increasing nursing care required and thereby adding to the burden of care. In hospital, these patients spend longer in bed and have longer lengths of stay. In a nursing home, these patients often consume more resources from carers, and are more prone to infections. Inadequate sedation may simply add to the disorientation and poor behaviour through drowsiness and disinhibition. Patients exhibiting signs of paranoia or extreme agitation may require acute sedation, using an antipsychotic such as haloperidol or one of the newer drugs such as olanzapine or risperidone (see Case Study 7.2).

Case Study 7.2

A 55-year-old woman with a diagnosis of Alzheimer's disease was admitted to a general ward after becoming unresponsive. She was mute with generalised increased tone, a temperature of 38°C and a mildly raised creatine kinase. She was taking haloperidol and the dose had recently been increased when she became disruptive whilst in respite care during a family holiday.

The haloperidol was stopped and her condition settled, with no cause for her pyrexia being found. A diagnosis of neuroleptic malignant syndrome was considered not proven, but the decision was made to avoid further exposure.

When she recovered she was very restless and would not sit in her chair. When left to wander she was at risk through inquisitive behaviour. She was constantly opening cupboards and interfering with equipment such as the cardiac defibrillator. She would frequently try to dance with frail patients, causing them to fall. Attempts to restrain her often produced a violent reaction.

An extra member of staff was assigned to walk with her and her behaviour became more manageable by diverting her attention away from critical situations without attempting to restrain her. The patient slept poorly, so the staff member was required 24 hours a day.

Attempting to restrain confused patients will often result in a breakdown in the patient–professional relationship, fostering paranoia and worsening disruptive behaviour. Alarms for seats or beds may help nursing staff to monitor the situation. In ideal circumstances, the patient should be allowed to roam in a safe environment. This is not usually possible in a general ward because of the wealth of critical areas the patient can invade, as illustrated in Case Study 7.2. Cot-sides for beds will not prevent confused patients from wandering. Instead, they simply provide an extra means of accidental injury.

It is important to recognise that many patients with dementia often exhibit a significant worsening of their cognitive function when acutely ill. The physician must therefore make every effort to exclude an acute, treatable pathology. Patients with dementia often present with very vague symptoms when suffering intercurrent illness, and a trawl of investigations including blood screen, urine culture, chest X-ray and ECG is quite acceptable for the patient with acute on chronic confusion. A review of medication is also mandatory. All drugs likely to have a negative effect on cognitive function should be discontinued, if possible.

It is not uncommon for the dementia to be undiagnosed. Very often a patient presents with an acute confusional state and only after careful discussions with family or carers does the history of increasing forgetfulness over several months become apparent. Personal experience suggests that relatives do not always equate confusion and forgetfulness. They often interpret confusion as an acute delirious reaction with altered consciousness and disruptive behaviour.

A common problem for the physician managing a patient with dementia in a general hospital is that the patient's cognitive impairment may hinder their treatment. This may be due to lack of ability to consent, or lack of compliance. A doctor in the UK is allowed to treat a patient 'in their best interests' if they are unable to consent to treatment.[19] This is rarely a problem where the proposed treatment is life-saving.

There is also the question of how to manage the patient who continually refuses to co-operate with treatment. Efforts should be made to gain the patient's trust and co-operation. In light of the patient's forgetfulness, it is usually advisable to involve the nearest relative or responsible carer in the discussion. This has the dual function of allowing the relatives to understand the situation and also allowing the physician to understand what the patient's philosophy was when they were well. In the UK, the law of consent makes it clear that if an adult patient lacks the capacity to consent, no one else may give or withhold consent on their behalf unless appointed by a court. Under such circumstances, the responsibility to give immediate life-saving treatment lies with the physician and not the family. For more complex decisions, the physician may need to consider taking legal advice.

It is also important for the physician to recognise that a diagnosis of dementia does not in itself indicate lack of capacity to consent. Consent requires the patient to understand the consequences of either accepting or declining medical advice. To assess this requires the doctor to evaluate the patient's understanding and ability to retain information about the issue requiring consent. The Department of Health guidelines for the UK require that any doctor should be able to assess capacity to consent, so this is not an issue solely to be assessed by psychiatrists.

If a patient lacks capacity to consent to medical investigations, the physician must take into account the consequences of forcing the patient to have the test. For instance, sedation or even anaesthesia might be required to carry out a CT scan if the patient is unable to co-operate. This would add a significant risk of morbidity, and perhaps a risk of mortality, to the procedure and judgements about the risks and benefits of the test would clearly need to take that into account.

At the extreme of refusal to consent, the patient may not take sufficient food and fluid to maintain their health. In such circumstances the physician should consider co-existent depression or paranoia, and may need to seek psychiatric advice. If there is no other treatable psychiatric condition, a detailed discussion with the family should be undertaken so that they understand the issues.

A more common problem in geriatric medicine is the patient with advanced dementia developing dysphagia. Dysphagia is perhaps more common in vascular dementia than Alzheimer's disease. A patient with dementia and dysphagia poses the difficult question of artificial feeding. Initially, attempts should be made to alter the consistency of food and supervise feeding. If this fails then the patient's individual circumstances should be carefully assessed, including discussions with the family about their views and whether the patient had previously expressed an opinion on this matter.

There is sufficient evidence showing that artificial nutrition by nasogastric or percutaneous gastrostomy (PEG) is associated with a higher incidence of aspiration and shorter life expectancy to indicate that artificial nutrition should only be instituted after careful consideration.[20] There is also evidence to suggest that offering appropriately thickened fluid and softened food in frequent small amounts is associated with weight gain, and this may be the most appropriate course of action.

For some patients the dysphagia requiring PEG indicates a very poor prognosis, with a UK study suggesting a 30-day mortality rate of 54%, rising to 78% at three months.[21] Under these circumstances, invasive procedures are unlikely to be in the patient's best interests. Informing relatives of the gravity of the situation is a very valuable part of the information exchange.

Finally, patients with dementia often cause difficulty when it comes to planning discharge. They require a more careful assessment of their ability to cope because of the unreliability of self-reported abilities. Patients with significant confusion require an objective assessment of their ability to carry out simple everyday tasks. If they live alone, their ability to manage safely in the kitchen should be assessed. They should be taken and assessed in their own homes to identify what risks they face on discharge. The occasion can be used to assess their orientation within their own home to help decide how much they appreciate their environment. Often the patient will perform better within their own home because of the familiarity of the surroundings.

If a home visit goes well, with no insurmountable safety concerns, carers and relatives may still be concerned about the patient's safety. Such concerns should be discussed because there may be issues that would not be identified on a home visit, for instance a patient who wanders out of their house at night.

Compliance with medication due to forgetfulness may also be an issue. Where this is a problem, attempts should be made to remind the patient. This can take the form of getting carers to give the medication, putting the medication in calendar packs and asking carers to monitor compliance and remind the patient if necessary, or even telephoning the patient to remind them to take their medication. If drugs have a narrow therapeutic index, e.g. warfarin, the need for the medication should be reviewed to ensure that the benefits of the treatment still outweigh the risks.

Key points

- Older people presenting with a history of gradual decline should have their cognitive function assessed routinely.
- People with undiagnosed dementia often present to the physician with another, unrelated condition.
- There is no evidence to support the cost-effectiveness of routine screening for the so-called reversible dementias in the absence of clinical indications.
- There are no controlled clinical trials to support treatment of an underlying cause of reversible dementias, but observational studies suggest improvement rather than cure.
- Patients with dementia in a general hospital often pose significant problems and are entitled to have access to appropriate expertise in their assessment and management.
- Clinicians should always consider capacity to consent to treatment of patients with dementia. Every patient with dementia should have their capacity to consent assessed because a diagnosis of dementia does not automatically imply a lack of such capacity.
- Dysphagia in patients with dementia requires a full multidisciplinary assessment
- Artificial feeding carries a high risk of morbidity and mortality in patients with dementia. Regular, small amounts of oral food and fluid of an appropriate consistency may be a more appropriate management plan.
- Patients with dementia should have an objective assessment of their ability to manage at home prior to discharge from hospital. Self-reported abilities may be unreliable.

References

1 Weytingh MD, Bossuyt PMM and van Crevel H (1995) Reversible dementia: more than 10% or less than 1% – a quantitative review. *Journal of Neurology.* **242**: 466–71.
2 Fox JH, Topel JL and Huckman MS (1975) Dementia in the elderly: a search for treatable illnesses. *Journal of Gerontology.* **30**: 557–64.
3 Clarnette RM and Patterson CJ (1994) Hypothyroidism: does treatment cure dementia? *Journal of Geriatric Psychiatry and Neurology.* **7**: 23–7.

4   Thompson WG and Freedman ML (1989) Vitamin B$_{12}$ and geriatrics: unanswered questions. *Acta Haematologica.* **82**: 169–74.

5   Siu AL (1991) Screening for dementia and investigating its causes. *Annals of Internal Medicine.* **115**: 122–32.

6   van Goor LP, Woiski MD, Lagaay AM *et al.* (1995) Review: cobalamin and mental impairment in elderly people. *Age and Ageing.* **24**: 536–42.

7   Gilbert GJ (1997) Cobalamin deficiency [Correspondence]. *Neurology.* **48**: 295.

8   Anon (1990) Vitamin B$_{12}$ deficiency and geriatrics [Comment]. *Acta Haematologica.* **84**: 108.

9   Bowie PCW, Corrado OJ and Waugh MA (1989) The prevalence of positive serological testing for syphilis among elderly hospital admissions. *Age and Ageing.* **18**: 407–10.

10 Boodhoo JA (1989) Syphilis serology screening in a psychogeriatric population. Is the effort worthwhile? *British Journal of Psychiatry.* **155**: 714–15.

11 Larson EB, Reifler BV, Sumi SM *et al.* (1986) Diagnostic tests in the evaluation of dementia: a prospective study of 200 elderly outpatients. *Archives of Internal Medicine.* **146**: 1917–22.

12 Bowie PCW, Corrado OJ and Waugh MA (1990) Screening for syphilis. *British Journal of Psychiatry.* **156**: 283–4.

13 McGlone J, Gupta S, Humphrey D *et al.* (1990) Screening for early dementia using memory complaints from patients and relatives. *Archives of Neurology.* **47**: 1189–93.

14 Kolbeinsson H and Jonsson A (1993) Delirium and dementia in acute medical admission of the elderly in Iceland. *Acta Psychiatrica Scandinavica.* **87**(2): 123–7.

15 Williams PS, Rands G, Orrel M *et al.* (2002) *Aspirin for vascular dementia* [Cochrane Review]. In: *The Cochrane Library, Issue 4.* Update Software, Oxford.

16 PROGRESS Collaborative Group (2002) Presented at: Annual Scientific Meeting of International Society of Hypertension, Prague, June 2002.

17 Qureshi KN and Hodkinson HM (1974) Evaluation of a ten-question mental test in the institutionalized elderly. *Age and Ageing.* **3**: 152–7.

18 Department of Health (2001) *National Service Framework for Older People.* DoH, London. Available from Department of Health, PO Box 777, London SE1 6XH.

19 Department of Health (2001) *Seeking Consent Working with Older People.* DoH, London. Available from Department of Health, PO Box 777, London SE1 6XH.

20 Finucane TE, Christmas C and Travis K (1999) Tube feeding in patients with advanced dementia. *Journal of the American Medical Association.* **282**: 1365–70.

21 Sanders DS, Carter MJ, D'Silva J *et al.* (2000) Survival analysis in percutaneous endoscopic gastrostomy feeding: a worse outcome in patients with dementia. *American Journal of Gastroenterology.* **95**: 1472–5.

8

The general practitioner's perspective

Linda Harris

Introduction

The National Service Framework for Older People[1] was published in 2001. In common with other NSFs, it is based around standards and charges local health and social care agencies with the task of putting in place a systematic and sustainable programme by which theses standards will be implemented. The NSF sets standards for the care of older people across health and social services. These standards apply whether an older person is being cared for at home, in a residential setting, or in a hospital. The NSF focuses on:

- rooting out age discrimination
- providing person-centred care
- promoting older people's health and independence
- fitting services around people's needs.

It specifically addresses those conditions which are particularly significant for older people and which have not been covered in other NSFs: stroke, falls and mental health problems associated with older age. But conditions such as stroke and dementia are not limited to older people, and the standards and service models will apply for all who need them, regardless of their age.

The programme of NSFs is part of the Government's agenda to improve standards and reduce unacceptable variations in health and social services. In the NHS, standards will be:

- *set* by the National Institute for Clinical Excellence and NSFs
- *delivered* by clinical governance, underpinned by professional self-regulation and lifelong learning
- *monitored* by the Commission for Health Improvement, the new Performance Assessment Framework and the programme of patient and service user surveys.

At present there are an estimated 700 000 people with dementia in the UK. The rise in the numbers of elderly people, especially the 'very old', means that GPs are finding themselves managing an increasing number of people with dementia. In Europe, dementia is more common than stroke in terms of both incidence and prevalence, but mental illness, especially depression and dementia, goes unrecognised in primary care.[2]

Ten years ago, the journal *Geriatric Medicine* surveyed 500 GPs from a random sample of 1500 readers and found that six out of ten GPs found Alzheimer's disease very difficult to manage and eight out of ten felt there were insufficient local resources to help them deal effectively with this group of patients.[3] Ten years have passed, but it has taken the publication of reports such as the Audit Commission's 'Forget Me Not'[4] (see Box 8.1) – an analysis of mental health services for older people in England and Wales – and subsequently the NSF for Older People in 2001[1] (Standard 7) for the true magnitude of the task ahead in implementing the mental health aspects of the NSF to be recognised by health and social care.

The age-related prevalence of dementia coupled with the increasing numbers of elderly people raises difficult questions about causes and treatment. However, in responding to the management of the problem, health and social commentators advocate a holistic approach that will help both sufferers and their carers to bear the *burden* of dementia.

Not surprisingly, it is the strengths of general practice as the patient's advocate and the gateway to services that make it so central to the care of this group of patients.

The role of the GP in the early stages of the disease

NSF 7.35: 'For older people with suspected dementia, early diagnosis gives access to treatment, allows planning for future care and helps individuals and their families come to terms with prognosis.'

People with dementia and those caring for them often first seek help from their GP. It is clear that the GP and primary healthcare team (PHCT) have a key role in the early stages of the disease, providing information, support and competent advice. The surgery should be a place where patients and their carers can come for information about local services, presented in a way that they can understand.

With the availability of effective treatments for dementia, it is crucial that an early diagnosis is made so that anti-dementia drugs are made available to those patients who meet the criteria for treatment published by NICE. Despite this, a number of trust and social services staff have expressed concerns over the delay in some GPs identifying mental health problems, with situations often reaching crisis point before specialist mental health services are alerted.

Box 8.1 The Audit Commission's report 'Forget Me Not: mental health services for older people'

The Audit Commission's main findings:

- Only half of carers are told what the problem is, or how dementia is likely to affect their relative in the future.
- Many GPs require greater support to help effectively.
- Whilst most GPs were trained in managing depression, half had not received any specific training in managing dementia and did not use any specific tests or protocols to diagnose it.
- Older people with mental health problems could get help at an earlier stage if specialist professionals give advice and support to GPs.
- Older people with mental health problems need a thorough assessment of needs, often best carried out at home, and access to a range of services. But many do not have access to all they need, often because most of the resources for specialist mental health services come from health agencies and go on hospital and residential care.
- People who would otherwise need residential care could live at home, if provided with flexible home-based care by joint health and social services teams.

The Audit Commission's recommendations include:

- GPs and other primary care staff should provide better information, support and competent advice for users and carers.
- Mental health professionals should provide more training and support for GPs and primary care teams.
- Provision should be balanced more in favour of flexible home-based services to provide support where it is needed.
- Health and social services should work together more effectively to share information about the care of individuals and to make better use of their joint resources.
- Commissioners of health and social care should have better information about the services they provide, to whom, and how well they are working.
- Users and carers should be involved in assessments and decisions about their care.

Getting GPs involved in treating the physical as well as the mental health needs of patients exhibiting early signs of dementia

NSF 7.37: 'Initial diagnosis of dementia involves ... carrying out a physical examination and investigations such as blood and urine tests.'

One of the challenges of working with older people is the frequency with which diseases present in a non-specific way. The only safe rule in practice is always to suspect underlying physical illness in old people presenting with psychiatric syndromes. History remains undeniably the most important way of gleaning information from the patient, but for completeness and in the case of an acute or chronic confusional state an increasing number of key people need to be consulted such as relatives, the warden, the home help, neighbours and district nurses.[5]

The causes of acute, subacute and chronic disease states are dealt with elsewhere in this book and there are a large number of physical conditions that produce the clinical features of dementia, such as restlessness, impaired concentration, emotional lability, behavioural deterioration, fear and anger. It is important that GPs conduct a careful assessment and medical examination and give such patients the benefit of the doubt as well as their knowledge, avoiding the all too common conclusion that dementia or senility is entirely to blame.

Once a diagnosis has been made, the primary aim is to ensure that any physical illness is treated as swiftly as possible, efforts are made to relieve physical discomfort and an early review of medication is made. Patients with confusional states related to physical problems often need help from specialists in both medicine and psychiatry of old age, and throughout the process information, advice and counselling for relatives will need to be provided by the GP.

Where dementia and depression co-exist

The prevalence of depressive disorder in patients with dementia is around 20%, and up to 10% of patients initially thought to have organic dementia are later diagnosed as having depression or depressive pseudodementia.[6]

For busy GPs, distinguishing between depression and dementia can be difficult. However, with careful assessment it is usually possible. Interestingly, the skills involved in unravelling this diagnostic conundrum illustrate the close relationship between depression and cognitive impairment and ensure that both of these important conditions are considered carefully in terms of the most appropriate assessment and management plan to be applied by the GP and PHCT. Box 8.2 lists some of the points to consider when managing patients with depression.

Box 8.2   Depression and dementia[6]

- Most patients with dementia are not depressed.
- Most patients with depression are not demented.
- Even when the two are found together, one usually predominates.
- Remember to assess both memory and mood in elderly patients.
- Depression often responds to antidepressants, even in dementia.

Cognitive impairment secondary to depression

Those elderly patients whose depressive illness is associated with profound psychomotor retardation, apathy, loss of motivation and slowed thought processes may perform poorly on bedside tests, suggesting a diagnosis of dementia. Many depressed elderly fail to keep up with basic self-care and lose weight, such that a dementia may be strongly suspected and a depressive illness may be overlooked.

Depression secondary to cognitive impairment

Depression in patients with dementia may have a psychological or organic cause. In early dementia, sufferers may retain sufficient insight to be distressingly aware of the loss of their valued intellectual abilities. Even more devastating will be the effects of their knowledge and understanding of the progressive nature of the disease, which is associated with increased suicide risk.

As dementia progresses, a patient's insight becomes impaired, leading to increasing disappointment, sadness and frustration at their failures at everyday tasks and loss of independence. In addition, organic brain disease may lead directly to low mood by affecting neuro-endocrine regulation or to an apathetic state that mimics true depression.

Factors leading to both depression and dementia

Various drugs and illnesses can cause both depression and cognitive impairment. One of the most important is alcohol, which whilst much less prevalent in the very old, causes low mood and cognitive functioning with the potential to cause permanent memory dysfunction and dementia.[7] It is important, therefore, to consider alcohol misuse in the elderly, and a simple questionnaire such as CAGE or the AUDIT questionnaire should facilitate further discussion in the consultation.[8] Drugs such as L-dopa, indomethacin, frusemide and steroids may all cause depression and delirium, especially in those with pre-existing organic brain disease.

Some diseases can precipitate either depressive or cognitive symptoms or both; these include Parkinson's disease, hypothyroidism and strokes. There are, of course, cases of coincidental co-morbidity where the two disorders occur together by chance and the longitudinal relationship evolves such that the earliest symptom of depression is dementia. This depression may merge later into dementia.

Tips on recognition and management of patients where the diagnosis between depression and dementia is unclear or where there is a combination of depression and cognitive impairment

The most important diagnostic aid is the history from both patient and where possible a reliable informant. Enquire about the onset and duration of symptoms and about other illnesses, drugs taken and alcohol. Certain features are linked more with depression or pseudodementia. These include:

- relatively short duration between onset and consultation
- previous psychiatric history
- a more precise date of onset of symptoms
- they are more likely to complain of poor memory and tend to be self-critical
- they are more likely to answer with 'I don't know' answers
- recent and remote memories are equally impaired.

Good management is reliant upon the GP or PHCT member using a standard assessment tool such as the abbreviated Mental Test Score, which is accurate at detecting dementia (see Box 8.3). Depression on the other hand is more easily overlooked, although a simple enquiry into the patient's mood perhaps coupled with a standard mood questionnaire such as the Geriatric Depression Scale[9] is

---

Box 8.3   Abbreviated Mental Test[15]

Each question scores one mark. No half marks. A score of 6 or less suggests dementia.
1 Age
2 Time (to nearest hour)
3 An address, e.g. 42 West Street, to be repeated by the patient at the end of the test
4 Year
5 Name of hospital, residential institution or home address depending on where patient is situated
6 Recognition of two people, for example doctor, nurse, relative, home help etc.
7 Date of birth
8 Year First World War started
9 Name of present monarch
10 Count backwards from 20 to 1

extremely useful in determining the true underlying cause and thereafter the most appropriate care plan.

It is important, therefore, to consider mood even in someone with established dementia, as depressive symptoms will often respond to antidepressants. It is important also to remember that even modest improvements in symptoms can make large differences to carers.

Sharing the diagnosis with patient and carer

NSF 7.39: 'Treatment of dementia always involves explaining the diagnosis to the older person and any carers and where possible giving relevant information about sources of help and support.'

Remember: patients and carers need to have the diagnosis explained to them and there should be regular opportunity for information as to how the disease or illness is likely to progress to be shared in a sensitive and collaborative way.

The challenges posed by attempts to maintain confidentiality and the autonomy of the patient

Many patients are resistant in the early stages to proposed interventions and changes in their routines and there are clear obligations for the GP and PHCT around patient confidentiality. Clearly, autonomy is to be encouraged, bearing in mind the limits of patients' abilities. Driving is one of the relatively few instances when it is appropriate for an official body to impose its judgement on both carer and patient.[10] In general, most decisions about management are best made by those most closely involved with the day-to-day life of the patient rather than by a committee or the courts. A balance must be struck between paternalistic care and a naïve attachment to the patient's overriding right to self-determination. When dealing with the sensitive area of fitness to drive, GPs will often refer to the regularly updated handbook published by the Driver and Vehicle Licensing Authority (DVLA) which contains helpful information and guidance.

For many relatives this will be their first experience of the illogicality and inconsistency of dementia, and whilst the professional will know that pre-emptive action before a crisis occurs will usually result in a better outcome and improved quality of life, all too often there is collusion, difficulties accepting the diagnosis and conflicts between the partners of dementing patients.

Ultimately, it is through open discussion of problems and possible solutions that optimum care can be achieved. Major management decisions can then be made collectively, by all members of the PHCT and the family, in consultation as much as possible with the patient. Occasionally, a consensus view is difficult to achieve. The GP is then ideally placed to act as a moderator, balancing the background knowledge of patient and family with his/her own experience.[11]

Managing the patient with a diagnosis of dementia when specialist services have to become involved

Once a specialist becomes necessary then the GP is often the professional called upon to make contact with the community mental health team who will then conduct a comprehensive assessment in the patient's home. By this time the GP should have performed a mental health assessment and will have looked carefully for underlying physical causes, including organising baseline investigations.

If patients are to benefit maximally and carers are to understand and be in a position to offer support then all the involved professionals need to exchange information and share decision making. Experience over the years has shown me that the actual membership of the team is less important than the systems the team members set up to communicate between themselves and with other relevant groups, such as the community psychiatric team and the local social work team.

By April 2002 the NSF demanded a single assessment process be introduced for the health and social care of older people and this must include an appropriate assessment of the patient's situation and the needs of people with a mental health problem.

Since the balance of provision of care is now in favour of home-based care, the GP must remain in close contact with the family and the community mental health team to track the services that are put in place and ensure that the patient and carer are receiving the services that meet their needs in accordance with the stage of the illness.

Primary care practitioners realise just how much the burden of care falls to the relatives. Relatives and carers put up with many problems with good grace and are worn down by others (see Box 8.4). They are central to the success of the policy of community care but the personal costs to them are great, and it is imperative that we support them.[13]

> NSF 7.51: 'Patients with complex mental health needs can and should be treated and supported in the community and wherever practicable at home.'

GPs have that key role of orchestrating the provision of diagnostic services, community support and institutional care of the highest standard. GPs feel confident in home care services if they are accessible and when they are provided sensitively and flexibly.

Frustrations are experienced where there is limited access to a multidisciplinary mental health team. The NSF demands that the core members of a specialist mental health service should include a consultant psychiatrist specialising in mental health problems in old age, community mental health nurses, clinical psychologists, occupational therapists and social workers, and that home care workers be trained in the management of mental health problems. It also prescribes a written care plan for service users on the care programme approach, but it is good practice to provide one for all patients so that the patient, their

---

Box 8.4   Problems associated with caring for older people with significant mental health morbidity[12]

Carers' problems – well tolerated
- Reduced social life
- Embarrassment
- Anxiety and depression
- Dressing
- Washing
- Urinary incontinence

Carers' problems – poorly tolerated
- Aggression
- Verbal abuse
- Wandering
- Faecal smearing
- Inappropriate urination
- Sleep disturbance
- Restless by day

---

carers and the healthcare providers all understand the management that has been planned.

GPs need to know that all of the above is in place and that in addition they can also access day-care facilities providing a range of stimulating group and one-to-one activities and also respite care, including emergency respite. Through this network, GPs can more confidently support and encourage carers to continue caring and co-operate with home-based models of treatment.

Managing the patient with dementia who lives alone

Luckily, the majority of Alzheimer's disease patients live with carers or have the benefit of carers' regular input. However, a small and significant minority live alone, which results in the potential for delayed diagnosis and a failure to track the deterioration in cognitive and physical functioning.

The Alzheimer's Disease Society and old age specialists have tried to encourage primary care-based 'over-75 health checks' in order to identify people with possible dementia who have nobody else to report their lapses of memory and difficulties with self-care.[14] This means going to the homes of those who have not attended the surgery lately, and including in the examination some form of cognitive test, such as the Abbreviated Mental Test Score.[15]

Sadly, despite the drive to engage more GPs and their PHCTs in the early detection and monitoring of patients who have dementia and live alone, evidence suggests that GPs, overburdened with the responsibilities of meeting the growing needs of all of their patients, will make no more house calls than they need to and rarely perform a cognitive test. It seems that they are sceptical of the benefits of early detection and fear the demands on their time. The whole system must acknowledge this and seek to engage as many GPs as possible in this task so that they can remain the focal point for care co-ordination.

The GP and the patient whose clinical condition is deteriorating

Finally, as the disease progresses, patients may no longer be in a position to cope at home and once again the GP may become involved in organising an admission to hospital or a bed where there is more intensive nursing care. GPs can and should advocate for maintaining as many people as possible in the community, provided that the psychiatric and behavioural problem does not preclude management in the community.

Hospital admission is sometimes unavoidable and provides an often much needed opportunity to holistically review the social care package and community care plan. Upon discharge of the patient, the GP is often faced with a revised community care plan and changes to the patient's medications. The post-discharge visit is therefore vital to update the GP records and ensure that GP and PHCT continuity of care is maintained.

Out-of-hours services are becoming increasingly sophisticated with respect to the care of older people with dementia. This is largely due to the development of care pathways supported by district nursing services and rapid response teams. Single assessment systems mean that increasingly a GP contacted out of hours can access a practitioner from rapid response, who will arrange for the patient to be supported either in their own home with additional support or arrange admission to a resource centre. The GP will usually need to visit and assess the patient to ensure that medical problems are identified, then a contribution to the patient's overall assessment of risk can be made and a treatment plan developed.

The development of intermediate care services means that increasingly primary care trusts (PCTs, see Box 8.5) are facilitating admission directly to residential and nursing homes. This requires a shift of resources in order to expand

---

Box 8.5 Primary care trusts

Primary care trusts are organisations that commission and provide health-care to a defined population. Most PCTs in England and Wales provide primary care, community and hospital-based services, and supporting services to a population of approximately 300 000. Many of the PCT's services will be delivered in partnership with other statutory and voluntary organisations. The trust is an employer and has a budget provided by the Department of Health that is the source of the majority (approximately 75%) of the heath spending for the population it serves.

the numbers of mental health specialists working in the community, to enable such homes to care adequately for highly dependent individuals.

Education and training for GPs and the PHCT: what do GPs want?

> NSF 7.45: 'Specialist mental health teams should work with primary care trainers to develop training in at least one screen for cognitive impairment, one depression screen and assessment of suicide risk.'

Surveys reported in the Audit Commission's *Forget Me Not*[4] show that over 50% of GPs report feeling insufficiently trained in the recognition and management of dementia. This is in stark contrast to the management of depression where around two-thirds feel sufficiently trained.

Training and support from, in the first instance, local specialist mental health teams have been highlighted as the way forward in engaging increasing numbers of GPs in the assessment process that leads to early diagnosis.

It is known that assessment scales aid the diagnosis of dementia by providing standard questions and a way of scoring them. They are useful in indicating the severity of cognitive impairment and are easily applied in the primary care setting. Despite this, the Audit Commission's surveys showed that fewer than half of the GPs were using specific screening tools or protocols to help diagnose depression or dementia.[4]

The NSF has tasked PCTs with the development and implementation of locally agreed protocols for the management of depression and dementia, but it will be the enthusiasm and willingness of local mental health professionals to provide training and guidance to GPs and primary care staff that will be key to successful engagement.

Primary care mental health leadership within PCTs and other developing networks, such as the National Institute for Mental Health, must aim to equip primary care staff with a basic understanding and awareness of mental health problems faced by older people and the relevant skills.

One excellent way of accessing GPs and the practice teams is to utilise protected learning time sessions, which are facilitated and funded through the PCTs and allow GP surgeries to close for training one half day per month. Local community mental health teams must be encouraged to approach practices to deliver training events, particularly those with a low referral rate. All practices must at the very least receive training in recognition and assessment, including the use of assessment scales for dementia and depression.

The promotion of the use of screening tools, such as the validated Mini-Mental State Examination and the Geriatric Depression Rating Scale, within a care pathway is the responsibility of NSF local implementation teams. PCTs must ensure that every general practice is using a protocol agreed with local specialist services to diagnose, treat and care for people with depression and dementia.

Training is known to reap rewards and there is strong evidence linking the provision of training and the value placed by GPs on early detection.[16]

The GP and information quality and clinical audit

The NHS Plan[17] emphasised the importance of the modernisation and expansion of computerisation in primary and secondary care. Clinical systems are designed and updated to keep pace with the technological revolution in healthcare and the ultimate goal, which is a comprehensive electronic patient record.

The 'over-75 health check' can easily be incorporated into a comprehensive electronic template, which can be populated by any member of the PHCT involved in the care of the elderly. The templates should be completed at least annually and information coded so that it can illustrate health trends and be used to monitor performance against targets.

Clinical governance departments of PCTs can assist practices to design clinical audits, using the information on their elderly care templates. Practices can track their progress in monitoring patients with a diagnosis coded as dementia, including medication checks and the recording of assessment scores such as the MMSE.

The GP and medicines management

The NSF has set targets for primary care around the review of medications for the over-75s on their lists. PCT's medicine management teams are tasked with ensuring that every GP offers a full medication review at least annually, with most GPs being encouraged, and where necessary supported, by the PCT to offer three- to six-monthly reviews for those patients taking over four medications. PCTs are working to increase the involvement of the community pharmacists in helping older people use their medicines appropriately.

GP practices can develop systems to help them meet this key milestone. Clinical computer systems and the maintenance of elderly care disease registers will enable them to audit their care and progress in this respect.

The gains for older people with mental health problems in reviewing medication are many, as they are the group most often in need of prescribing advice and support and most likely to be using four or more drugs. Regular review by the GP will improve the quality and cost-effectiveness of prescribing and avoid waste. Good practice in this area will reduce adverse reactions to drugs and the risks of suicide associated with medicines. The review provides an opportunity for the GP to ensure that the medicine is providing the intended effect and detect any medicine-related problems. It will also help to avoid the trap of leaving patients with dementia on potent drugs prescribed for short-term sedation or the management of behavioural disturbance.

Promoting the health of the patient with dementia

Good medicines management is one very important way that a patient's health can be promoted. However, all older patients, regardless of cognitive functioning, have the right to access the benefits of modification of the risk factors for disease, even if their mental health is deteriorating as part of a dementia-type illness.

Primary care is seen as the main way to access mainstream health promotion and disease prevention programmes. The PHCT, in particular the practice nurses, can advise patients and carers on the most appropriate and meaningful actions around primary and secondary prevention, addressing mainly chronic disease management, problems relating to mobility such as prevention of and managing the consequences of osteoporosis, and access to the annual flu vaccination campaigns.

It is worth remembering that multi-infarct dementia is more common than was previously estimated and should be preventable through programmes of stroke risk factor prevention.

The surgery can also signpost families and carers towards programmes for increasing physical activities, and encourage the pursuit of hobbies and interests, the 'keep warm, keep well' campaigns and healthy eating.

Conclusions

I hope I have demonstrated how the GP and practice team can become useful companions to patients with dementia on their journey of care. By walking the clinical path *with* the patient, the GP will remain in the best position to support the range of needs of both patients and their families.

Such complexity needs to be managed through co-ordination between health and social care through integrated teams of services. Efforts to ensure effective information sharing, working alongside that patient and a willingness to consult and/or visit them regularly means that the GP will continue to be central to the care planning of patients with dementia.

With the ever-increasing demands being placed on primary care to deliver the growing number of NSFs, a strong commitment is required of the practice team, supported by the PCTs to prioritise the standards of the NSF for Older People.

Education and training from local specialist mental health teams will help to build bridges and equip PHCT members with much needed skills and tools to help them undertake their most important role, that of early detection and monitoring.

By becoming involved proactively in the multidisciplinary management of dementia, the GP and practice team will be rewarded. Potential benefits include being able to competently deal with the increasing needs of patients in a timely, evidenced-based manner, with the added bonus of seeing the carers (so often also your patients) gain the tangible benefits of integration into mainstream primary care services.

Carers need to be empowered to cope, and patients need to know that their GP practice will support and facilitate their right to early assessment and equal access to the full range of physical and mental health services they deserve.

Key points

- GPs and nurses in the primary care team are recognised as having a crucial role in early, accurate diagnosis of dementia and its successful management.
- Training for GPs and the PHCT in dementia management is an important area for PCTs to focus on, and vital if attitudinal change and improvements in the recognition and management is to occur. This should concentrate on professional role, good practice strategies, early and accurate diagnosis, use of cognitive assessment tools, coping mechanisms for difficult behaviours and support resources.
- Many resources are required in dementia care, including clinical expertise from the doctor and an up-to-date, wide-ranging knowledge of local and regional resources. Any shortfalls in resource awareness will disadvantage the patient and their family. In the case of dementia, the caring, interested GP is often best placed to oversee care and identify and plug any gaps or faults in provision of care.
- NICE guidelines highlight the role of cholinesterase inhibitors in the management of dementia patients whose Mini-Mental State score is less than 12. GPs need to be aware of care pathways which enable access to specialist memory clinics.

References

1   Department of Health (2001) *National Service Framework for Older People*. DoH, London.

2   Jorm AF and Jolley D (1998) The incidence of dementia: a meta-analysis. *Neurology*. **51**: 728–33.

3   Grace J (1993) Alzheimer's disease: your views. *Geriatric Medicine*. **23**(1): 39–41.

4   Audit Commission (2000) *Forget Me Not: mental health services for older people*. Audit Commission, London.

5   Eccles J and Wattis J (1988) Underlying physical causes of confusion in the elderly. *Geriatric Medicine*. **18**(4): 55–63.

6   Rao R, Dening TR, Brayne C *et al.* (1997) Suicidal thinking in community residents over eighty. *International Journal of Geriatric Psychiatry*. **12**: 337–43.

7   Black DA (1990) Changing patterns and consequences of alcohol abuse in old age. *Geriatric Medicine*. **20**(1): 19–20.

8   (2000) Managing the heavy drinker in primary care. *Drug and Therapeutics Bulletin*. **38**(8).

9   Yesavage J (1986) Geriatric Depression Scale (GDS): recent evidence and development of a shorter version. *Clinical Gerontology*. **9**: 165–73.

10 Oppenheimer C (1991) Dementia and driving. In: R Jacoby and C Oppenheimer (eds) *Psychiatry in the Elderly*. Oxford University Press, Oxford.

11 Jones RG (1993) Ethical and legal issues in the care of demented people. *Reviews in Clinical Gerontology*. **3**: 55–68.

12 Argyle N, Jestice S and Brook CPB (1985) Psychogeriatric patients: their supporters' problems. *Age and Ageing*. **14**: 355–60.

13 Levin E, Sinclair I and Gorbach P (1989) *Families, Services and Confusion in Old Age*. Avebury, Aldershot.

14 World Health Organization (2002) Diagnosis and management of dementia in primary care. *Guidelines: Summary of Clinical Guidelines for Primary Care*. **16**(2): 164–6.

15 Qureshi K and Hodkinson M (1974) Evaluation of a 10-question mental test of the institutionalized elderly. *Age and Ageing*. **3**: 152–7.

16 Renshaw J, Scurfield P, Cloke L *et al*. (2001) General practitioners' views on the early diagnosis of dementia. *British Journal of General Practice*. **51**: 37–8.

17 Department of Health (2002) *The NHS Plan*. DoH, London. www.doh.gov.uk/ nhsplan/nhsplan.htm

9

The role of the nurse in the assessment, diagnosis and management of patients with dementia

Richard J Clibbens and Dianne Lewis

Introduction

Nurses are in a powerful position to influence the care of people with dementia for good or ill. The richness of the nursing contribution to care can be compromised or destroyed where insight, knowledge or communication skills are lacking. The care and support of people with dementia is predominantly carried out in a community setting. Care is often led or delivered by families, neighbours, friends and unqualified care workers. Interventions by professionals must acknowledge this and do nothing to imperil or destroy existing, often complex, networks of support.

Assessment

Nurses have a vital and often central role in the assessment of people with dementia. The range of settings and opportunities for nurses to positively engage in these processes of assessment is diverse, ranging from general health screening with older people in primary care, through to specialist memory assessment clinics and myriad other clinical and care situations. Nurses working in general hospital settings and residential or nursing homes, for example, may be the key professional or named nurse co-ordinating the care of older people, in settings which are recognised to include a high prevalence of dementia.[1]

The nursing role in assessment and diagnosis may be in providing a unique nursing perspective or in co-ordinating multidisciplinary assessment in addition to completing the core elements of a comprehensive person-centred assessment. The value of this contribution has not always been recognised:[2]

Nursing people with dementia has low status because it is perceived as an area involving much 'routine' care and little technological expertise.

(Cantley, p. 233)

The potential roles and influence of nursing in the assessment of people experiencing dementia have been identified to include:

- being the 'main support' person
- independently assessing the person at home, in clinic or hospital
- history taking from the person and family
- administering psychological tests
- carrying out joint assessments with colleagues.[3]

The Royal College of Nursing (RCN) Assessment Tool for Nursing Older People[4] has been identified as a potentially useful core framework for the nursing assessment of an older person's needs.[1,3] People who are or may be experiencing dementia clearly require a full global nursing assessment in addition to a specific focus on their unique experience of dementia.

In assessment, account must be taken of the relationships and family dynamics as carers may resist interventions which are interpreted as threatening to their 'normalisation'.[5]

A systematic approach to assessment is required in which strengths and positive factors are identified as well as hazards which pre-dispose people to risks in certain circumstances.

Parsons, p. 134

While assessment scales can form a useful component of assessment, for example of baseline cognitive function, they are still only a part of the whole picture of that person's experiences and are not usually diagnostic in their own right.[6]

The National Service Framework for Older People[1] identifies that completion of a physical examination, including the completion of blood and urine tests, is an essential component of the initial diagnosis of dementia. Nurses are increasingly able to either instigate or administer these test procedures in their clinical practice.

Whether at the level of health screening in primary care, during hospital admission or in residential care settings, nurses, in collaboration with medical colleagues, must ensure that an appropriate initial physical assessment is carried out for people who may be experiencing dementia (see Box 9.1). This must include screening to exclude underlying physical illness or delirium. Agreed protocols for cognitive screening and initial assessment can assist in appropriate screening for, and detection of, dementia in primary care. This can enable appropriate joint working with, or referral to specialist mental health services for people with dementia.

Box 9.1   Baseline investigations for dementia[7]

- Full blood count
- Erythrocyte sedimentation rate
- Vitamin B_{12} and folate
- Thyroid function tests
- Urea and electrolytes
- Calcium
- Liver function tests
- Glucose
- Blood tests for syphilis, serum lipids and HIV are optional
- Simple urinalysis should be performed
- ECG/chest X-ray if indicated by significant cardiovascular system, or respiratory system, features
- CT scan, when indicated by signs and symptoms of the illness

---

Sharing the diagnosis

Alzheimer's Disease International[8] have described the shock of a dementia diagnosis, emphasising the value of good, accurate information in assisting to resolve some of the anxiety at this time for the person and their family. Nurses can utilise their roles in a range of health settings to provide support, education and information at such critical times as these in the journey of dementia, for both the person and their family.

The nursing contribution to diagnosis sharing in dementia is often of vital importance.[3] Nurses are often well placed to have identified the person's wishes with regard to diagnosis disclosure over a period of time. This may include the identification of any conflict of interests in diagnosis sharing with the person's family. For example, a person experiencing memory impairment may fear being assessed as unfit to hold a driving licence following receipt of a dementia diagnosis, while their family may have concerns for their driving safety and view a diagnosis as enabling this situation to be managed.

Alzheimer's Disease International[8] have identified that listening to the person's 'story' of the development of dementia is the most important element of diagnosis. Nurses are often the members of the multidisciplinary team best placed to elicit and record the person's story, fulfilling a key role in accurate assessment and diagnosis. Nurses can combine this key role with a unique individual representation of that individual and their personal history, translating the assessment process into a vehicle for recognition of the individual and validation of their personal and unique identity in the presence of dementia. At a time of potential great stress and anxiety, the nurse may be able to recognise the potential strategies and reactions of the person with dementia, who may appear resistive to the process of diagnosis and assessment.[9] Life-story books can be useful in enabling people with dementia to retain and consider their individual identity in the midst of many changes.[10]

Interventions

Assessment is often the first of many interventions. Whether engaged in assessment and care planning in the earlier stages or further through the person's individual journey of dementia, the nurse can have a key influence on how this is experienced by the person and their family:[11]

> The key principles which emerge are concerned with ensuring that practice is undertaken within a person-centred, values-based approach which sustains a focus on positive action and which actively works to ensure that dependency and negativity is always minimised. These principles are equally applicable across all stages in the process, across all professions and across service settings.
>
> (Stanley and Cantley, p. 122)

Significant differences may exist between professional notions of assessment and diagnosis and that of the person with dementia and their family.[12] In recent years, a number of studies have begun to explore the experience of dementia from the perspective of the person, and now people with dementia themselves are describing their experience of dementia in research studies exploring diagnosis disclosure.[13]

There are potential conflicts of interest in responding to the expressed views and wishes of the person with dementia and that of their carers or family. Identified differences of opinion must be objectively recorded within the assessment process, clearly identifying who has expressed them.

Assessment of behaviour

The potential difficulties experienced by a person with dementia in social settings, such as a hospital ward or residential home, can lead to behaviour which may be described as 'challenging' or 'disturbed'. This may be related to a whole range of factors related to how that individual relates to people, their physical environment and also their internal perception and understanding of what they are experiencing. The potential loss of normal social inhibitions, problems in recognising people and their roles, or difficulty understanding what is expected from them are some potential challenges for the person with dementia in relating to those around them. Behavioural changes and disturbance experienced by the person with dementia may have significant impact on carers and be a key element in placement decisions and planning the provision of care.[14]

The many potential losses experienced by a person with dementia entering a formal care setting, such as familiarity, independence, security, companionship or orientation, can potentially be profoundly distressing and associated with behaviour labelled as disturbed, especially in the presence of any impaired communication abilities. It may be difficult for the person with dementia to retain a sense of their unique identity in the presence of potential loss of skills and social roles, combined with anxiety or fear for their future.[15]

In assessing the behaviour of people experiencing cognitive impairment, the nurse will need to obtain an objective assessment of exactly what is occurring. This can be achieved by observing and accurately recording the following elements of what is often described as 'disturbed behaviour':

- what were the **A**ntecedents (what was happening immediately before the behaviour occurred)

- what was the **B**ehaviour (objective description of what the actual behaviour was, not interpretations of what the behaviour may mean)

- what were the **C**onsequences of the behaviour (what were the outcomes for the person and others).

This information can be collected over time across the 24-hour care period and evaluated in the context of that person's unique identity and life history. It may be useful to consider a range of questions:

- Does the behaviour represent the psychological, physical or emotional expression of pain or distress?

- Is the person's previous ability to verbally communicate altered in the presence of dysphasia?

- Is the person experiencing sensory deficits?

- Does the behaviour occur at a particular time?

- Is it in response to a particular situation or person?

- Is it related to communication between the person and others?

- Is it related to care-giving interventions?

- Is it related to external stimuli in the environment?

- Is the person fulfilling a psychological/emotional/physical need by this behaviour?

It may often be possible to identify periods of time where a person needs more support. If, for example, a person with dementia in a medical ward becomes distressed each time their visitors leave, can their sense of possible isolation, loss or abandonment be made more bearable through engaging in a social intervention with nursing staff on the ward at the point at which their family depart?

With their detailed and often intimate care contact with people with dementia in formal care settings, nurses can utilise their knowledge of the person to plan individualised care and interventions to minimise many potential causes of reported behavioural disturbance.

In relation to risk management with people with dementia, careful assessment and observation is essential.[16] The person's true ability to function in their own environment must be assessed and not their ability to function in the potentially disorientating environment of a hospital ward. This is essential when planning for discharge and the provision of care packages. Nurses acting as key workers for people with dementia have a vital role to ensure that effective multidisciplinary assessment has taken place at the right time and in the right environment to facilitate maintaining the person's optimum functioning.

The word 'dementia' may instil a fear into the person to whom it is applied, that they are somehow necessarily less capable. Nurses have a vital role in ensuring that the person with dementia's right to consent to care and treatment is maintained. Where a person may lack capacity with regard to any element of independent decision making in relation to their health and social care, this must be formally expertly assessed.[17] Clearly, each individual will experience dementia differently, with differing rates of progress of the condition and differing retained strengths and experienced losses. Too often the term dementia can still be interpreted to suggest some form of automatic loss of capacity. As nurses we must question 'who' is deciding 'what' is in the person's best interests, and on what basis.

The nursing contribution to the management of people suffering from dementia has, according to Menzies,[18] complied with the theory of the biomedical nature of dementia, as it has a positive advantage of allowing nurses to retreat into emotional non-involvement when lacking personal resources available to deal properly with people with dementia.

Person-centred care

The exhortation to deliver person-centred care in modern health and social services does not co-exist easily with the existing pressures and organisational and educational designs. A key role for nurses is to influence strategic thinking and planning to address this incongruity.

A nursing focus of care must be 'to assist sufferers and relatives to find meaning within the illness experience and to assist them to preserve, even during the final deterioration of the patient, a notion of personhood'[19] (see Box 9.2).

The extensive work related to personhood and dementia by authors such as Kitwood has, according to Adams,[21] done much to set dementia and it's care within a moral framework which attributes value to people with dementia.

Box 9.2   Six criteria for personhood[20]

1 Consciousness (particularly the capacity to feel pain)
2 Reasoning
3 Self-motivating activity (i.e. renewable behaviour driven from within)
4 The capacity to communicate
5 The presence of self-concept
6 Self-awareness

Nurses have a unique opportunity and responsibility to lead and influence the formal and informal care team in the establishment of person-centred care. Regardless of the arena, a nursing diagnosis must build upon a skilled, informed and sensitive interpretation of assessment. This, in conjunction with a clinical diagnosis, must generate clear and specific statements which identify the person and their family's actual and potential needs and retained strengths and abilities.

It is essential to recognise the potential for multi-pathology to be present in older people and the rapidly changing balance between delirium and dementia in planning and evaluating interventions and care (see Box 9.3 and Case Study 9.1).

Box 9.3 Effective individual nursing intervention in dementia care

- The identification of strengths and needs by debate with the person, carers and relevant others.
- The establishment of a nursing diagnosis built upon accepted models, relevant to client group and context.
- The documentation of information in a rational and accessible manner. The use of information technology where appropriate and respecting confidentiality.
- The prioritisation of actions from a patient and carer perspective.
- The establishment of evidence-based practice in response to the individual's strengths and needs.
- The evaluation of interventions against stated goals.

Case Study 9.1

Mrs P has been diagnosed as experiencing dementia. Her care is delivered by her husband in their own home with the support of the community psychiatric nurse (CPN). The CPN receives a call from Mr P: there has been a significant change in Mrs P's behaviours and routines. She has been up all night, is resistive to help, anorexic, agitated and tearful, all of which, according to her husband, were sudden in onset. On the arrival of the CPN, Mrs P looks unkempt and agitated, her husband is visibly distressed, and even the pet dog appears anxious and does not offer his usual friendly greeting.

The skilled intervention of the nurse includes:
- initial reassurance and support
- observation of present interactions
- ensuring Mrs P is in a safe environment, that other members of the care team support Mrs P while discussions take place with Mr P to:
  - clarify the duration of change

> – identify and exclude, where possible physiological causes for the delirium
> – request the assistance of the GP for further refinement of the diagnosis.
>
> The nurse identified these possible actions in response to the assessment:
> - treatment in Mrs P's own home for physiological problems
> - an agreement to review in 24 hours
> - agreed additional support for a time-limited period
> - an urgent outpatient review by Mrs P's consultant
> - transfer to hospital or assessment unit for further assessment and diagnostic procedures.

Admission to an acute hospital setting has the potential to create a major crisis for a person experiencing dementia and their supporters. It is often a perilous passage through a busy and noisy accident and emergency (A&E) department where patients and their relatives are required to be expert and articulate historians to assist in diagnosis and planning. The initial contact may be with professionals with a limited understanding of dementia. Inappropriate gathering or recording of information at this point can have life-changing consequences for the person and their carer. It is at this first hospital encounter that the nurse, working in an institution, can drive and influence others in the delivery of person-centred care for the patient and their supporters (see Box 9.4).

Box 9.4   Person-centred care[22]

- Respect for personhood
- Valuing interdependence
- Investing in care-giving as a choice

Liaschenko,[23] cited in Nolan,[24] indicates three broad types of knowledge to inform nursing practice:

- *Case knowledge*: this comprises biomedical disembodied knowledge of a particular condition, for example stroke illness.

- *Patient knowledge*: this is best viewed as the 'case in context'. In other words information about a person's social circumstances, level of support and so on, to provide a better understanding of the impact of the illness and resources which can be mobilised.

- *Person knowledge*: this is based on understanding the 'biographical life' which for Liaschenko comprises three components:
  - *agency*: the capacity to initiate meaningful action
  - *temporality*, which is related to an individual's pattern of life rather than 'clock time'

  – *space*, in terms of how an individual relates to their physical, social and political environments in order to create a sense of 'belonging somewhere'.

Skilled intervention can begin to elicit all three of Liaschenko's[23] described 'types of knowledge', but acknowledges the requirement for trust and time to pursue this and the potential conflict in a situation where the primary aim is to cure a condition and move a person out.

Diagnostic and therapeutic interventions in A&E departments may stimulate behaviours in the patient which have been previously unseen or concealed by relatives. The ensuing concern and distress must be recognised and managed. Transfer to a ward area, therefore, may deliver a patient and family at their most vulnerable into an already busy clinical area. Interactions at this time may set inappropriate benchmarks upon which future actions and relationships are built. Tolson *et al.*[25] describe the potentially threatening nature of an acute ward environment and the feeling of worthlessness generated in both patients and visitors.

Tolson *et al.*[25] also identify that acute nursing care is at its best when delivered in tandem with recognition of the special needs of the person with dementia. The recognition and planning of care for a person with dementia must be clearly translated into effective and consistent care delivery. Tolson has identified the lack of recognition of, or recording of, assessments relating to cognitive impairment in documentation within acute hospital settings.

Risk management

A lack of understanding, explicit recording and debate about behaviours which may be challenging and distressing or constitute a risk to the person with dementia themselves or others, can imperil person-centred care. The growing number of older people with delirium or dementia who require care or support in all settings demands creativity in information collection and utilisation. Table 9.1 and Boxes 9.5 and 9.6 illustrate an approach to explore a nursing perception of challenging or risk-creating behaviours and activities in cognitively impaired patients in an acute general setting, which, in the pilot area, resulted in the creation of documents and formed the foundation of work to understand the causes of such behaviours and improve a patient-centred management of them.

Table 9.1   Documentation relating to domains of behaviour and ensuing care management

RISK IDENTIFICATION TOOL (PILOT)

Name...Ward ....Date................................

Domain	Risk identified	Date	Behaviours to warrant risk identification may include:
Wandering off or around the ward			• Leaving the ward without prior arrangement • Apparently aimless wandering • Wandering to opposite sex side of ward
Personal safety			• Risk of self-harm • Moving furniture • Slipping on urine or faeces inappropriately voided • Falling due to poor mobility • Falling out of bed or climbing over cot rails
Interfering with others – patients, visitors and/or nurses			• Banging bed rails • Invading others' personal space • Mistakenly taking others' belongings • Noisy at night • Distracting nurses from specific activities, e.g. medication • Attracting attention of other visitors, causing them distress
Aggressive behaviour aimed at others			• Shouting loudly in an aggressive manner • Aiming punches or kicks at others • Gesticulating in a manner causing distress to others
Poor nutritional status			• Throws food on floor • Delusional beliefs regarding food • Removing artificial feeding devices (e.g. nasogastric tubes/IVs)

Loss of personal dignity	• Inappropriate removal of clothing in presence of others • Passing urine inappropriately • Soiling own clothes • Being laughed at by others for their behaviour • Wandering to opposite sex side of ward • Deterioration in personal hygiene habits • Inappropriate expression of sexuality
Escalation of risk at particular times	• Meal times • Medication time • Visiting times • Night time
Validity and consistency of accuracy of communication with others	• Forgetting interactions with medical team • Forgetting interactions with nursing and therapy team • Inaccurate recall about fluid and food intake • Mismanagement of own property and valuables

Other comments:

Box 9.5   Recommended good practice in the management of people with cognitive impairment

Problem: Risk associated with cognitive impairment.
Aim: To reduce risks.

Plan:
• Always address the patient in the manner they prefer.
• Involve friends and family in the assessment process.
• Complete the risk assessment documentation.
• Involve medical staff in assessment and management.
• Allow the patient time to get settled into the environment.
• Always explain in detail what is happening and why.
• Ensure that any special needs are catered for (e.g. sensory or physical disability).
• Establish what may calm the patient when they are distressed or agitated.
• Establish usual routines and habitual ways of behaving.

- Keep visitors informed concerning medical and nursing care. This intervention should be 'proactive'.
- Reduce agitation.
- Establish level of observation as appropriate.
- Always record and report on behaviour at the end of each shift.

Box 9.6   Positive approaches to reducing agitation

Positive approaches to reducing agitation may include:
- good light to ensure good visibility of environment
- quiet atmosphere
- familiar objects in the patient's immediate environment
- clear orientation signs indicating day room, toilets, etc.
- liaison with medical staff to review prescribed medication and exclude any possible underlying physical cause.

The concept of 'expert' patient and 'expert' carer, which may be presented in the form of patient/carer diaries or explored by skilled nursing intervention, provides the opportunity for nurses and nursing to be the champions of person-centred care.

The development of new roles/designs of care delivery provides enormous opportunities for skilled nurses to lead person-centered care (see Case Studies 9.2 and 9.3). Nurse-led rehabilitation units, nurse-led intermediate care facilities and outreach mental health teams – providing clinical support, assessment, advice and education to primary, secondary, intermediate and long-term care settings – are seen as a significant contribution to the development of integrated mental health services demanded by the National Service Frameworks.

Case Study 9.2

Mrs S has an established diagnosis of dementia and has been supported in her own home by a complex network of lay and professional carers. The daughter of Mrs S leads family input. There have been increasing concerns about the safety of Mrs S as she is becoming increasingly frail and is discovered on the lounge floor at 8 a.m. by her daughter on her 'routine call' to give mum her breakfast, prior to commencing work. Mrs S is cold, shocked and has obvious pain in her leg/hip. An ambulance is called. Mrs S has fractured her femur and is 'fast-tracked' on arrival at the hospital, using an integrated care pathway designed to meet the immediate needs of a person suffering from a fractured neck of femur. Post-operatively, Mrs S is withdrawn, drowsy and reluctant to take fluid or food. The briefest details were recorded prior to surgery. The nurse who is leading the care of Mrs S now begins to establish 'who this person is', recording information from Mrs S where possible and from her daughter. The nutritional assistant has asked about her favourite food and drinks.

Her daughter states: 'They reminded me about her glasses, I had forgotten in the rush. They explained about the anaesthetic, pain tablets, change of environment and trauma before and after admission and how they may have affected Mum. This made me feel better. I thought I had "lost my Mum". The care plan was there for Mum and I to see, and the physiotherapist was so patient and knew Mum soon forgot her advice and gently reminded her. They asked us to bring family photographs for Mum's locker, and I wrote down what time I would visit where she could see it. Mum had always been a very quiet person and since her illness was unlikely to instigate a conversation, but even on this busy ward I felt they cared about her, and valued her enough to find out about her and I never felt she was "abandoned in the corner".'

Assessment of Mrs S's post-operative condition acknowledged that she may not demonstrate discomfort, pain, thirst, hunger, bladder or bowel problems in 'normal' ways and skilled interventions ensured that these were identified and managed. Rehabilitation processes acknowledged her short-term memory loss, and skilled discharge planning built upon retained strengths and well-established support networks and ensured discharge was timely and well supported.

Case Study 9.3

Mrs D has been an inpatient in a hospital-based assessment unit for people with a diagnosis of dementia. Mrs D was admitted at the request of her CPN who had been supporting her care in the community with a complex care package. Mrs D had suffered a series of falls and her cognitive function and self-care abilities had deteriorated over the past two months. Mrs D, her family and GP were involved in and agreed with the decision to admit. Skilled, nurse-led assessment, physiological investigations, medication review and full assessment by the multidisciplinary team then contributed to a case conference with Mrs D and two family members present. The CPN assisted Mrs D and her family to describe events prior to admission. The nurse leading Mrs D's care within the unit presented the results of the inpatient assessment. The agreement was reached by all that Mrs D required 24-hour care in a residential setting.

Mrs D was considered to have the cognitive capacity to make an informed decision by her consultant. In an uninformed setting this would be seen as almost an end stage. To the skilled team, recognition that admission to a residential home is a significant life event to the person and her family will ensure that selection of the home, support of Mrs D, her family and the care-home team, provision of excellent information and continued support as each assumes new roles in life will be a challenge met by nursing leadership and liaison.

Combating ageism

The principles of good practice are generic and clearly indicated in the Department of Health's NSF for Older People[1] and *The Essence of Care*.[26] Demographic change results in increasing numbers of people with dementia being present in the community, acute hospital settings and specialist dementia assessment and care units, while the private health and social care sector provides growing levels of longer-term dementia care. Endemic ageism, in conjunction with changing work and public agendas give added resonance to the 'six senses' as described by Nolan (see Box 9.7).[24]

Box 9.7   The six senses[24]

1 A sense of security

For older people: Attention to essential physiological and psychological needs to feel safe and free from threat, harm, pain and discomfort.

For staff: To feel free from physical threat, rebuke or censure. To have secure conditions of employment. To have the emotional demands of work recognised and to work within a supportive culture.

2 A sense of continuity

For older people: Recognition and value of personal biography. Skilful use of knowledge of the past to help contextualise present and future.

For staff: Positive experience of work with older people from an early stage of career, exposure to role models and good environments of care.

3 A sense of belonging

For older people: Opportunities to form meaningful relationships, to feel part of a community or group as desired.

For staff: To feel part of a team, with a recognised contribution, to belong to a peer group – a community of gerontological practitioners.

4 A sense of purpose

For older people: Opportunities to engage in purposeful activity, the constructive passage of time, to be able to achieve goals and challenging pursuits.

For staff: To have a sense of therapeutic direction, a clear set of goals to aspire to.

5 A sense of fulfilment

For older people: Opportunities to meet meaningful and valued goals, to feel satisfied with one's efforts.

For staff: To be able to provide good care, to feel satisfied with one's efforts.

6 A sense of significance

For older people: To feel recognised and valued as a person of worth, that one's actions and existence is of importance, that you 'matter'.

For staff: To feel that gerontological practice is valued and important, that your work and efforts 'matter'.

The impact of dementia on the person themselves, their family and teams of carers can be devastating. The massive changes in health and social care delivery, design and expectations can be viewed as creating similar responses in nursing and care staff. Perhaps this shared experience of learned helplessness will have positive outcomes for all.

The wider role of nurses in dementia care

The NSF for Older People,[1] and *The Essence of Care*[26] both provide clear indications of service expectations. Within these frameworks there is a growing role for nurses as they guide, direct and monitor care, and enable patients and carers to be fully involved with care decisions and care delivery (see Box 9.8).

The clinical governance framework demands an advanced level of skills and knowledge and the ability to recognise and manage the changing nature of people requiring care and support. The increasing knowledge and changed expectations of some service users and their protection within legal frameworks, combined with growing numbers of frail elderly people who are vulnerable to abuse, illustrate the complexity of service delivery and the requirement for person-centred care.

The nursing contribution to healthy ageing is a complex and profound phenomenon. Evidence-based practice, with a patient-centred focus, can be directed and monitored by the nurse, who can exploit to the full their relatively high level of direct patient contact and their advanced assessment and interdisciplinary working skills.

Service development and new roles

There is now a developing interest across the NHS in designing integrated service protocols and care pathways for people with dementia, with nursing staff often locally leading and implementing these initiatives, working with local agencies and multidisciplinary teams. Memory clinics are becoming a core part of

---

Box 9.8 Nursing input

Strategic influence
- Care environments – site and design
- Skill mix and staffing levels and the creation of new roles
- Selection of models of care
- Development of pathways of care
- Documentation design
- Structures for interfaces

Operational influence
- Person assessment
- Care planning/evaluation
- Guidance of, and referral to, others
- Role modelling
- Medication selection, administration and monitoring
- The delivery of the essential elements of care
- Support of, and interaction with, family and lay carers
- Advocacy with and for the person experiencing dementia and the detection and management of abuse in its varying forms
- Conflict resolution within lay and professional networks
- The planning, support and monitoring of discharge, including contributions to the care programme approach
- Outreach and education

---

many local older people's mental health services[1,27] and nurses are often core members of these teams (see Box 9.9). Moniz-Cook *et al.*[28] have described the use of individualised programmes for people in the earlier stages of dementia, which incorporate counselling for losses, reinforcement of coping strategies, crises prevention advice and memory management programmes, tailored to the specific needs of the individual.

Box 9.9 An innovative nursing role within a memory clinic

The Wakefield Memory Clinic (South West Yorkshire Mental Health NHS Trust) provides an initial assessment undertaken by a dedicated community memory clinic nurse, who negotiates a suitable assessment date and time, visiting the person at home to complete an initial baseline global assessment, including completion of the Mini-Mental State Examination[29] and where appropriate the Geriatric Depression Scale: 15 Item,[30] or Hospital Anxiety and Depression Scale (HADS).[31] Information is provided to the person and their family on the memory clinic assessment process and a direct booking is made for an appointment with the nurse consultant or medical staff at the clinic for more detailed cognitive assessment, if appropriate.

The national Audit Commission,[32] has identified the need for local services to review their practice and procedures for explaining to older people or their carers what problems they may face and how these may be positively managed in the presence of dementia.

The Mental Health Foundation[33] have supported six two-year pilot projects with local services providing information, advice and support for people in the early stages of dementia.

The NSF for Older People'[1] identifies that mental health nurses are 'core members' of a specialist mental health service, who will be working in integrated multidisciplinary teams with psychiatrist, psychologist, therapy and social work colleagues. Nurses are increasingly taking on specialist roles, providing outreach or liaison services from specialist older people's mental health services to nursing and residential homes.

The starting point for good quality nursing assessment of an older person is an identification of what exactly is to be assessed and why. Department of Health guidance on the single assessment process for older people[34] identifies the usefulness of specific assessment tools in identifying specific health conditions such as cognitive impairment. Assessment scales used should be valid, reliable and culturally sensitive. Overview assessment tools for use with older people, such as EASY-Care,[35] are designed for use by any front-line health or social care professional, providing prompts for more specific detailed assessment, including for cognitive impairment or depression. The RCN assessment tool,[36] has also been identified to provide a holistic nursing assessment of the older person's needs.

Ethical practice

The person with dementia's life story or 'narrative' enables identification of the person's past life, biography and autobiography, and recognition of other important figures in that person's life.[37] This information can be crucial in informing the application of any notions of consent or capacity in the care and treatment of that person. Providing quality information at the right time, and identifying the person's 'unique biography', is the basis for good nursing assessment. A partnership model between the person with dementia and the professionals,[27] can be placed at the core of nursing roles and interventions for diagnosis, assessment and care planning with people with dementia and their carers.

People with dementia are able to express their views and wishes,[2] and the nurse must strive to ensure that this is clearly demonstrated within any process of assessment. Engaging in the assessment of people with dementia, as in all areas of nursing practice, requires a consideration of the ethics of our action or inaction. Do we assume our role gives us a right to ask the person questions about their life?[38] In seeking the person's consent to the process of assessment, the aims and objectives must be clearly stated. Do we always clearly identify why the questions are being asked and what they will be used for? If not, are we acting truthfully and honestly? In completing nursing assessments with someone experiencing dementia, we must be aware of the potential that we are using our position of trust with the person we are assessing to somehow 'trick' them into full disclosure of their experiences, thoughts and plans, without informing them of the potential consequences of this for their future care and treatment.

Acting 'ethically' in any given nursing situation with a person with dementia will require the nurse to pay attention to conflicts of values within themselves and between themselves and others.[39] In caring for people experiencing dementia, the nurse is frequently faced with the dilemma of balancing the person's 'best interests' with their personhood and right to self-determination. Increasingly, as nurses we find it easy to talk of 'recognising the person' not the illness and of ensuring the person consents to care interventions, but truly achieving this in our practice can be a significant challenge in dementia care.

Key points

Nursing input:
- has powerful potential for positive *or* negative outcomes
- can either prevent *or* underpin negative and inappropriate labelling
- can gather and utilise essential information, using their skills to separate fact from opinion
- can be the therapeutic presence for people experiencing dementia and their families
- can contribute to conflict resolution within families at a time of great vulnerability.

References

1 Department of Health (2001) *National Service Framework for Older People*. DoH, London.
2 Cantley C (ed.) (2001) *A Handbook of Dementia Care*. Open University Press, Buckingham.
3 Royal College of Nursing Institute (1999) *Nursing in Memory Clinics: resource pack*. Royal College of Nursing, London.
4 Ford P, Blackburn S, Heath H *et al.* (1997) *Introduction to the RCN Assessment Tool for Nursing Older People*. Royal College of Nursing, London.
5 Parsons M (2001) Living at home. In: C Cantley (ed.) *A Handbook of Dementia Care*. Open University Press, Buckingham.
6 McKeith I and Fairburn A (2001) Biomedical and clinical perspectives. In: C Cantley (ed.) *A Handbook of Dementia Care*. Open University Press, Buckingham.
7 Royal College of Psychiatrists (2002) *'Forgetful But Not Forgotten': assessment and management of dementia by a specialist service*. Presented at ARM, Jersey, 2002. Available at www.rcpsych.ac.uk
8 *World Alzheimer's Day Bulletin* (2001) Alzheimer's Disease International, London.
9 Keady J and Gilliard J (2002) Testing times: the experience of neuropsycholo-

gical assessment for people with suspected Alzheimer's disease. In: PB Harris (ed.) *The Person with Alzheimer's Disease: pathways to understanding the experience*. Johns Hopkins University Press, Baltimore, MD.

10   Woods B (1999) Younger people with dementia: psychosocial interventions. In: S Cox and J Keady (eds) *Younger People with Dementia: planning, practice and development*. Jessica Kingsley, London.

11   Stanley D and Cantley C (2001) Assessment care planning and care management. In: C Cantley (ed.) *A Handbook of Dementia Care*. Open University Press, Buckinham.

12   Keady J and Gilliard J (1999) The early experience of Alzheimer's disease: implications for partnership and practice. In: T Adams and C Clarke (eds) *Dementia Care: developing a partnership in practice*. Churchill Livingstone, Edinburgh.

13   Wilkinson H (2002) *The Perspectives of People with Dementia: research methods and motivation*. Jessica Kingsley, London.

14   Woods R (1999) Psychological 'therapies' in dementia. In: R Woods (ed.) *Psychological Problems of Ageing: assessment, treatment and care*. John Wiley & Sons, Chichester.

15   Cheston R and Bender M (1999) *Understanding Dementia: the man with the worried eyes*. Jessica Kingsley, London.

16   Marshall M (1997) *State of the Art in Dementia Care*. Centre for Policy on Ageing, London.

17   British Medical Association and the Law Society (1995) *Assessment of Mental Capacity: guidance for doctors and lawyers*. BMA, London.

18   Menzies-Lyth I (1988) (cited in Adams) *Containing Anxiety in Institutions*. Free Association Books, London.

19   Jenkins D and Price B (1996) Dementia and personhood: a focus for care? *Journal of Advanced Nursing*. **24**: 84–90.

20   Warren M (1973) (cited in Jenkins and Price) On the moral and legal status of abortion. *The Monist*. **57**(1): 43–61.

21   Adams T (1996) Kitwood's approach to dementia and dementia care: a critical but appreciative review. *Journal of Advanced Nursing*. **23**: 948–53.

22   Mulrooney CP (1997) *Competencies Needed by Formal Care-givers to Enhance Elder Quality of Life: the utility of the 'person and relationship-centred care-giving (PRCC) trait'*. 16th Congress of the International Association of Gerontology, Adelaide.

23   Liaschenko J (1997) Knowing the patient. Cited in Thorne SE and Hays VE *Nursing Praxis: knowledge and action*. Sage, Thousand Oaks, CA.

24   Nolan M (2000) Skills for the future of the humanity of caring. *Nursing Management*. **7**(6): 22–9.

25   Tolson D, Smith M and Knight P (1999) An investigation of the components of best nursing practice in the care of acutely ill, hospitalised older patients with coincidental dementia: a multi-method design. *Journal of Advanced Nursing*. **30**(5): 1127–36.

26   Department of Health (2001) *The Essence of Care*. DoH, Leeds.

27   Keady J (2001) *Early Intervention in Dementia: a review of service responses*. Presented to the *Journal of Dementia Care* Conference, Dublin.

28 Moniz-Cook E, Agar S, Gibson G *et al.* (1998) A preliminary study of the effects of early intervention with people with dementia and their families in a memory clinic. *Aging and Mental Health.* **2**(3): 199–211.

29 Folstein M, Folstein S and McHugh P (1975) 'Mini-Mental State': a practical method for grading the cognitive state of patients for the clinican. *Journal of Psychiatric Records.* **12**: 189–98.

30 van-Marwijk H, Wallace P, de-Boc G *et al.* (1995) Evaluation of the feasibility, reliability and diagnostic value of shortened versions of the Geriatric Depression Scale. *British Journal of General Practice.* **45**: 195–9.

31 Zigmond AS and Snaith RP (1983) The Hospital Anxiety and Depression Scale. *Acta Psychiatrica Scandinavica.* **67**: 361-70.

32 Audit Commission (2002) *Forget Me Not: developing mental health services for older people.* Audit Commission, London.

33 Mental Health Foundation (2001) *Dementia Advice and Support Services: an update from the Mental Health Foundation.* Mental Health Foundation, London.

34 Department of Health (2002) *The Single Assessment Process: assessment tools and scales.* DoH, London. www.doh.gov.uk

35 Sheffield Institute for Studies on Ageing (1999) *EASY-Care Elderly Assessment System.* Sheffield Institute for Studies on Ageing, University of Sheffield.

36 Royal College of Nursing (1997) *Guidelines for Assessing Mental Health Needs in Old Age.* RCN, London.

37 McCormack B (2001) *The Person of the Voice: narrative identities in informed consent.* Presentation Abstract of the *Journal of Dementia Care* Conference, Dublin.

38 Barker PJ (1997) *Assessment in Psychiatric and Mental Health Nursing: in search of the whole person.* Stanley Thornes, Cheltenham.

39 Johns C (1995) Framing learning through reflection within Carper's fundamental ways of knowing in nursing. *Journal of Advanced Nursing.* **22**: 226–34.

10

The occupational therapist's perspective

Mary Duggan

Introduction

Occupation is a word in common usage that has a highly specific meaning to the occupational therapy profession. Kielhofner[1] defines human occupation as 'doing culturally meaningful work, play or daily living tasks ... in the contexts of one's physical and social world'. Occupational therapy is directly concerned with the individual's ability to meet their personal needs for engagement in activity, and the demands placed on them by their social and physical environment. The role of the occupational therapist is to work with individuals whose ability to meet these needs is impaired by illness or disability.

We exist within a complex matrix of social networks, physical environments, occupations and activities. They contribute to the maintenance of our identity. Dementia cannot be fully understood unless it is seen in the context of the individual's physical, social and occupational setting and their experience of it. This chapter explores:

- the impact of dementia on engagement in activity
- the assessment of occupational performance
- occupational therapy interventions.

The impact of dementia on engagement in activity

The Model of Human Occupation[1] is founded on the belief that meaningful occupation is central to our well-being and that human occupation can best be understood as a dynamic system that involves:

- physical and social environments
- habituation
- skills
- personal causation.

Physical environment

The physical environment tends to become less accessible for us as we age. Decreasing energy and loss of physical fitness makes us less mobile. Places where we like to spend our time or that we need to visit become less easy to get to or to move about in. The physical environment does not just relate to places and spaces. It also involves the materials and tools that we use to perform activities. We select some of these because of their functionality, but many of the objects that we surround ourselves with are chosen as an expression of our personalities.

Dementia may initially produce disorientation in place, making it harder for the individual to make their way about unfamiliar places. In the later stages of dementia, the individual may lose the ability to recognise familiar places (see Case Study 10.1) and possessions. The physical environment, far from being a place of security and comfort, may become strange and threatening.

Case Study 10.1

Louise began to turn up at the local police station almost every day. No longer able to recognise her own home, and frightened by finding herself in what seemed to be a strange house, she took the logical course of going to the police. She was confident that they would take her home, which of course they did. It did not take long for the police to realise that she needed help and to refer her to specialist services.

Social environment

We belong to a varied social network: family, friends, colleagues, acquaintances; people who provide the interaction that we enjoy and the services that we need. The process of ageing tends to diminish the social environment through reduced mobility and bereavement.

The impairment of short-term memory experienced in the early stages of dementia may lead to forgetting the names of familiar people. The embarrassment that this produces may make the person with dementia less willing to seek out social contact, beginning a gradual process of social withdrawal. As the dementia progresses, the individual may experience increasing difficulty with memory and with work-finding. The loss of communication skills contributes to difficulty in maintaining social relationships. The person may increasingly withdraw from challenging situations. Family and friends are likely to find communication with the person with dementia becoming more and more frustrating, as their conversation becomes repetitive and focused on past events. In the later stages of dementia, the individual may lose the ability to recognise familiar people, which is in itself a profound form of bereavement. The ability to initiate and maintain social contact becomes increasingly reduced.

We primarily experience ourselves as individuals through our interaction with others. Loss of this ability means that it becomes progressively harder for the person with dementia to maintain a sense of self, let alone self-worth.

Skills

Occupational behaviour is enabled by a wide range of physical, cognitive and interpersonal skills. Dementia is characterised by a gradual impairment of skills that may manifest in increasingly deteriorating memory, loss of attention span, reduced intellectual performance, communication difficulties and loss of judgement and capacity for abstract thought. In the later stages there may also be progressive and significant loss of physical functioning. The loss of skills results in an increasing inability to engage in purposeful occupational behaviour. In addition to this, it is likely that through an honest desire to reduce risk, the carers of the person with dementia deliberately reduce the range of activities that the individual can engage in, thus further eroding their ability to practise and maintain skills.

Habituation

Each of us has a repertoire of life-roles, and this role-set plays a large part in our sense of identity. Often, when meeting someone for the first time, we ask them what they do. Our role-set naturally changes as we move through life, including roles related to family, friends, work, study, community involvement and leisure activity. It tends to reduce as we get older. This loss of roles is linked to factors already mentioned: retirement, increased infirmity, loss of mobility, a reduced social environment. Every role has some value to us, and the loss of a valued role can lead to loss of self-esteem, and contribute to loss of identity.

Our ability to function effectively within our role-set is influenced by the skills that we have, and the behavioural routines that we develop. The loss of skills, described above, sets in train a vicious spiral: the individual becomes less able to engage in roles, and their reduced engagement brings with it a corresponding loss of opportunity to use and maintain skills. In addition, the loss of a particular role means a loss of the routines that support it, and therefore loss of some of the structure that enables us to make sense of our lives. Routines are dependent on our ability to remember them, and therefore may be lost as the individual's memory deteriorates. However, encouraging and supporting the person with dementia to maintain their roles and routines may be a major factor in maintaining their skills, engagement and independence.

Motivation

Personal causation is the extent to which we feel more or less competent or skilled at particular activities. Based on our experience of success, it influences our choice of activity or occupation, and produces the drive to engage in activity. It is affected by the values that we place on activities and our personal interests. Any reduction in the opportunity to experience skill, competence and mastery is likely to lead to a loss of motivation to engage in activity.

The loss of skills that is a major feature of dementia will inevitably result in the person with dementia experiencing failure in activities at which they were previously competent or even highly skilled. This contributes to the increasing spiral of withdrawal and disengagement.

Key points

- Dementia impairs the ability of the individual to function within their normal physical and social environment.

- Dementia is associated with progressive loss of roles and the routines that sustain them.

- Dementia is associated with loss of physical, cognitive and social function.

- Dementia is likely to reduce the individual's expectation of competence.

- People with dementia are treated differently to others.

Assessment of occupational performance

The term 'holistic' may be casually used in reference to assessment processes. It is perhaps more important in the assessment of the person with dementia than in any other clinical area that the assessment is genuinely holistic. This involves determining the impact of dementia on all aspects of the individual's life and experience. The contribution of occupational therapy is to assess the impact of dementia on an individual's occupational function and performance, and the Model of Human Occupation[1] (described above) gives a framework for this. The areas that should be assessed include:

- the individual's ability to perform required and desired activities within their normal physical and social environment

- the extent to which the individual's physical and social environments support or impede their functioning

- the roles that the individual wishes or needs to engage in

- the ability of the individual to maintain the routines that support these roles

- the skills demanded by roles and routines, and the extent to which the individual possesses these skills

- the individual's motivation or disposition towards required and desired activities, roles and routines, and their expectation and experience of competence.

There is no universal assessment that covers all of these. However, it is possible to assemble a battery of assessment tools and approaches that will provide a comprehensive evaluation of the needs, capabilities and aspirations of the person with dementia. The therapist should not make the assumption that dementia precludes the use of assessments that require verbal response, such as semi-structured interviews. Assessment should combine both observation and interview where possible. Any observation of task performance will only be fully meaningful if carried out in the setting in which the individual would normally perform that activity.

Occupational Performance History Interview II[2]

Originally developed as a generic measure of occupational performance, this semi-structured interview has been modified to match it more closely to the principles of the Model of Human Occupation.[1] It explores:

- the roles that make up an individual's lifestyle

- the ways that the individual organises and uses their time

- critical life events

- the individual's occupational environments, including home, productive activity and leisure, and taking into account the physical and social aspects of those environments

- the factors that influence choice of activity

- the individual's life story.

The assessment is summarised into three rating scales (each four-point):

- the Occupational Identity Scale: the extent to which the individual has goals, values, interests and expectation of success

- the Occupational Competence Scale: the extent to which the individual is able to engage satisfactorily in occupational behaviour

- the Occupational Behaviour Settings Scale: the extent to which the individual's physical and social environments support their choice of activity, and the extent to which chosen activities match their interests, abilities and personal resources.

Although this assessment seems lengthy on initial inspection, it can be broken down into modules and used over an appropriate period of time. It provides a rich picture of the things that an individual wants and needs to do, and the barriers to effective occupational performance. The authors state that it is suitable for adults who can reflect on and talk about their life history, including people with mild to moderate dementia.

Assessment of Motor and Process Skills[3]

The Assessment of Motor and Process Skills (AMPS) is designed to assess how an individual's motor and process skills affect their ability to carry out activities of daily living (ADL). The assessment is based on the observation of the individual carrying out selected daily living tasks from a specific range. The AMPS allows the individual to choose tasks that are meaningful to them and can be carried out in any relevant setting.

- Motor skills – the 'observable, goal-directed actions that the person enacts during the performance of ADL tasks to move oneself or the task objects'. Related to posture, mobility, co-ordination and strength.

- Process skills – the 'observable actions of performance that the person enacts to logically sequence the actions of the ADL task performance over time'. Related to attention, concept formation, organisation, planning and ability to adapt.

The tasks are calibrated according to their relative difficulty. In addition, each rater is given a calibration factor to adjust the raw scores in order to eliminate bias arising from rater severity. Recent research[4] indicates that the AMPS is able to distinguish between cognitively well people and people with dementia. The assessment analyses occupational performance and identifies actions that are not carried out effectively.

Pool Activity Level Instrument[5]

The assessments described above enable the therapist to identify the occupations, roles and routines that are important to the individual, and to gauge the extent to which motor and cognitive impairment may reduce or prevent engagement in meaningful activity. The Pool Activity Level (PAL) Instrument closes the loop, as it were, by enabling the identification of the developmental level that a person with dementia is at, and suggesting how activity can be structured to support continuing engagement in that activity. Based on an understanding of developmental processes, the PAL check-list uses the following developmental levels:

- Planned activity level – the individual is able to work towards task completion, but may need assistance with problem solving.

- Exploratory activity level – the individual can carry out familiar tasks, but is likely to be more interested in the experience of being engaged in activity rather than in the end result. They may need assistance in sequencing the activity.

- Sensory activity level – the individual is focused on immediate physical sensa- tion. At this level, people need assistance to perform simple tasks, and these tasks should give the person plenty of opportunity to experience a range of sensations.

- Reflex activity level – the individual may not be aware of their environment or of physical sensations. Movements that occur are not purposeful, but are in reflex to stimuli. Activities at this level will involve direct sensory stimulation, introducing a single sensation at a time.

The PAL Action Plan enables the therapist to identify activities that the indivi- dual is likely to be motivated to take part in, and describes in some detail how to structure that activity to maximise its effectiveness. The PAL is a highly effective tool for multidisciplinary care planning – it enables staff and carers to structure all of the activities that the person with dementia takes part in to ensure that engagement is maintained, and that activity is meaningful and a positive experi- ence.

Assessment of risk

There is great concern, rightly so, with the assessment of risk. Thom and Blair[6] describe the role of occupational therapy in identifying actual risks to the indivi- dual through the use of functional assessment based on observation and inter- view. They stress the importance of fully engaging with both patient and carers in this process. They acknowledge the tension that is present between risk prevention and the rights of the individual to take risks, and argue for a balance between risk and quality of life (see Case Studies 10.2 and 10.3).

Case Study 10.2

Annie was admitted to hospital because of concerns about her leaving her house and 'wandering'. In casual conversation, she began to reminisce about her earlier life, especially during World War II. She had always loved boats, and sailing. She was one of the people that risked their lives piloting small craft across the Channel to evacuate soldiers from the Dunkirk beaches. Now, some 50 years on, she was faced with the prospect of not being allowed to take any risks at all. This conversation caused the whole team to re-evaluate their attitudes towards Annie and risk, and certainly gave a completely different sense of proportion.

Case Study 10.3

Adam had been admitted to hospital because he was a high suicide risk. He knew that he had dementia, and hated the thought of living with it. He also desperately wanted to go home. The team worked very carefully with

---

Adam and his family, and came to the agreement that, while there would be a risk of him harming or even killing himself, this was outweighed by his wish to be at home. The care plan that supported his discharge from hospital provided daily, supportive contact that enabled the team to monitor his mood closely and sensitively. He was able to remain in his own home for a further 18 months before having to move into long-term care.

Of course, it is vital to be aware of the risks, and to carry out an assessment of the potential and actual impact of those risks on the individual. Thom and Blair[6] suggest, based on the literature reviewed, that the following areas should be considered:

- physical risks – cuts, falls, impaired mobility

- ability to operate household appliances safely

- personal risks – self-care, nutrition, medication compliance, continence, dressing

- coping with the outdoor environment – getting lost, going out at night, driving, shopping

- general risks – financial management, risk of being abused, home security, dealing with emergencies, communication ability, smoking, alcohol abuse.

In addition to risks of accidental self-harm described above, the risk of deliberate self-harm should not be ignored. In the earlier stages of dementia, the individual may well have insight into their illness. As with any progressive and indeed terminal illness, the individual is likely to question whether or not they wish to continue to live. Thoughts of suicide would not be unusual, and may be acted on.

Intervention

There is an argument that occupational therapists who work with people with dementia tend to focus their energies on functional assessment, and specifically on risk management. In a discussion of the role of the occupational therapist in continuing care settings, Perrin describes '... the craft of the occupational therapist, who must impose order upon the chaos of pain, disruption and dysfunction by the artful manipulation of occupations'.[7] It is vital that the occupational therapist not only identifies the barriers to occupational performance, as described above, but also uses a range of interventions to enable the individual with dementia to continue to engage in meaningful and purposeful activity, and to live as independently as possible in the least restrictive environment compatible with agreed levels of safety. The interventions used traditionally involve:

- modification of the physical environment

- modification of the social environment
- the use, modification or adaptation of purposeful activities or occupations.

Dementia is a progressive condition, and therapeutic intervention may move along a continuum from rehabilitation or re-ablement to adaptation and compensation with an overarching focus on maintaining engagement and personhood. Perrin and May[8] argue that the traditional rehabilitative approach, which has an ultimate goal of withdrawing support and increasing independence, is ineffective in the context of dementia care. They suggest that an understanding of the inter-relationship of occupation and well-being is of central importance, and that a 'state of "wellness", rather than of "health" is a more appropriate goal'.

Environmental modification

It is important that the individual's physical environment supports them in carrying out the activities that they need and want to do. The most significant environment is the individual's home and its surroundings. The therapist has a responsibility to guide the individual and their carers in eliminating unnecessary risk from that environment, but equally has a responsibility to ensure that the home remains a place where the individual can take part in meaningful and valued activity (see Case Study 10.4). There are obvious interventions: removing loose rugs that increase the risk of falls, reducing clutter to present a less confusing environment and ensuring that the materials and equipment needed for chosen activities are easy to locate.

Case Study 10.4

Mary was in the early stages of the dementia process. The Assessment of Motor and Process Skills enabled her therapist to look at the coping strategies that she was already using, and to tap into them. Mary kept her washing machine in the garage, and would often put clothes in but then forget about them. The AMPS indicated that she used visual cues to remind her of tasks. Her therapist suggested that each time she put clothes in to wash, that she left the box of soap powder out on the kitchen counter. This reminded her that she needed to go back and put the clothes in the dryer. This was a much more meaningful and effective coping strategy for Mary than a written list would have been.

Modifying the social environment is, perhaps, less obvious. The person with dementia may have become increasingly socially isolated. If this is due to lack of confidence in leaving the house, or loss of the ability to make their way to social venues, they may simply need assistance with transport. If they are finding it difficult to engage in activities, the therapist may need to consider introducing them to environments where these activities can be structured to support participation. Perhaps the most significant aspect of modifying the social environment is the work that may need to be carried out with the person's carers. This involves not only educating them about the nature and implications of dementia, but also involving them in the assessment process so that they have a clear picture of the person's ability as well as disability. The therapist can then explore the ways in which carers can continue to encourage and support the person's involvement in activity (see Case Study 10.5).

Case Study 10.5

Janet developed Korsakoff's syndrome while still in her mid-forties. She was admitted to hospital in an acutely confused state; she was confabulating, she had difficulty distinguishing between her dreams and waking experiences, and she was frightened about being in hospital. The OPHI II assessment (see p. 139) showed that productive activity was of great significance to her. She had given up a very responsible career because of the increasing deterioration of memory and cognitive functioning that she was experiencing, and was no longer engaging in any activity that was relevant to her and her needs. With encouragement, she chose to cook a meal, something that she would do on her return home. Her therapist used this to establish rapport, and also to give Janet a much needed experience of success. Janet began to show rapid improvement. The therapist worked with the team and Janet's family to help her to establish a more meaningful and satisfying routine. Her partner ran a small business, and agreed to give Janet some simple clerical tasks to do. She needed step-by-step instruction, and a huge amount of support from him, but this enabled her to re-establish a valued routine. She became happy and confident. She stopped drinking, and knew what coping strategies to use to avoid re-admission.

Activity modification

The core tenet of occupational therapy is that meaningful activity is central to our well-being. Perrin,[9] in a study using the dementia care mapping instrument developed at the University of Bradford by Kitwood, Bredin and others, identified that older people with dementia who are in long-term care spend much of their time unoccupied. There is a strong argument that the failure to provide opportunity for activity, whether this is in the context of a residential care setting or the person's own home, constitutes a form of abuse of people with dementia.

Therapists working with people in the early stages of dementia are likely to focus their energies on maintaining routines, skills and the individual's participation in activities and occupations of their choice (see Case Study 10.6). In the later stages of dementia, especially where the individual is functioning at the reflex or sensory levels described in the PAL tool, the meaningfulness of an activity may not always be apparent to the therapist (see Case Study 10.7). Careful observation and dialogue with carers may help the therapist to make an activity more meaningful and satisfying.

Case Study 10.6

Adam was an active man in his mid-fifties when he began to show signs of cognitive impairment. He still retained a degree of insight, and found it difficult to come to terms with the prospect of a progressive illness. This led to his hospitalisation as a suicide risk. On the ward, he showed a range of behavioural problems. The OPHI-II showed that routine was deeply significant. He had spent many years in the armed forces, and still had a very rigid daily structure. He talked with great pride about his past achievements; he had been a skilled leader and was highly respected. He was very clear about what he wanted: to return home, to be able to go for walks, to make himself drinks and snacks. In the ward setting, his own rigid personal routines clashed with the ward routines, leading to Adam expressing his frustration through 'difficult' behaviour. The therapist designed Adam's care plan around his routines, accompanying him on walks and encouraging him to make drinks for himself in his own room. These routines enabled the team to establish a package of support at home that was highly successful. Again, all of the interventions were timed to fit in precisely with his routine, and focused on checking that he was still maintaining his routine safely and successfully. Eventually, Adam needed to go into long-term care. The team helped him to make a smooth transition by finding a home that was able to create a care programme around his routines and activities. He still goes out with a member of staff for a daily run.

Case Study 10.7

Freddie began the multi-sensory session by crawling about on the floor. He often did this on the ward. He was giving the impression of being very busy, and concentrating hard on what he was doing. The therapy assistant suggested that he might be sweeping up. She gave him a brush, and he proceeded to sweep the entire floor, with great satisfaction. Here, the therapy assistant helped him to engage in an overtly purposeful activity. Sometimes, Freddie liked to stand at the old-fashioned wash-tub. He needed two people to help him to maintain his balance. He would enjoy pushing and pulling the scrubbing board back and forth. While there was no apparent external meaning to this activity, Freddie would focus on it for long periods of time. He was working. In fact, the only way to persuade him to rest was to suggest that it was time for a tea break. In this instance, it did not matter that the therapist did not understand the meaning of the activity; Freddie did.

There may also be an argument that when working with people in the later stages of dementia, where the focus of activity is on stimulating the senses and maintaining social contact, the nature of the activity is more important for staff and carers. Working with an individual who can give minimal feedback is tiring. Here, it is vital to have a wide range of activities that can be engaged in for as long as the individual's attention span allows, and that avoids monotony for all concerned. The occupational therapist can play a vital role here in suggesting suitable activities and also showing how to structure or modify them to enable the individual to engage. The concept that Perrin and May[8] describe as the 'bubble' can inform practice. This bubble is the boundary beyond which the person with dementia cannot perceive their surroundings. The bubble shrinks progressively. In this phase, the work of the therapist is one of reaching out, making and maintaining contact, through whichever activity and medium works in that moment. The goal of occupational therapy, and indeed of the multiprofessional team working with people with dementia, is ultimately to maintain the individual's sense of self, and most importantly their sense of being a valued person (see Case Study 10.8).

Case Study 10.8

The Orchard is a particularly lively and happy place. It provides day treatment, respite and continuing care for people with severe dementia. The building is designed to provide a non-restrictive environment. The only areas not accessible to the residents are the kitchen and the clinic. The day is filled with a mixture of organised and spontaneous activity. Objects that are designed to stimulate the senses are left around in the various rooms, and residents pick them up and use them at will. Therapists, nurses and care assistants work together to design individual plans of care. They use the PAL tool as a multidisciplinary assessment to gauge how best to structure activities for each person. The range of activities that they use is limited only by their imaginations. Some activities are simple, everyday tasks. Some use multisensory equipment. Behavioural problems, which are so often expressions of frustration, are few. If someone wants to wander around the building, then that is what they do. If someone needs assistance to do this, assistance is given. No one in that building is not a part of the care team and does not get directly involved with the residents.

Key points

- Dementia impairs the ability of the individual to engage in meaningful occupation.
- Occupational therapy assessment of the person with dementia should encompass their ability to perform the activities required by their roles and environment, the extent to which their physical and social environment supports their engagement in activity and their motivation towards activities and occupations.

- Assessment should draw on a range of approaches, including the use of standardised assessments, observation and interview. Therapists should strive for balance between the management of risk and the rights of the individual to take risks.
- Therapeutic interventions with the individual with dementia may involve:
  - modifying the physical environment so that it supports engagement in occupation
  - modifying the social environment so that it supports engagement in occupation
  - modifying or adapting purposeful activities or occupations to support engagement.
- The overall focus of assessment and therapeutic intervention with the person with dementia should be to maintain their engagement and sense of self.

Acknowledgements

I am grateful to Katie Barker for the Case Studies, and to Jane Currie, Programme Manager and James Waplington, Clinical Manager (both at the Older People's Services, South West Yorkshire Mental Health Trust, Wakefield, UK) for their support.

References

1   Kielhofner G (1995) *A Model of Human Occupation: theory and application* (2e). Williams & Wilkins, Baltimore, MD.
2   Kielhofner G, Mallinson T, Crawford C *et al. Occupational Performance History Interview II*. Model of Human Occupation Clearing House. www.uic.edu/hsc/acad/cahp/OT/MOHOC
3   Fisher AG (1999) *Assessment of Motor and Process Skills* (3e). Three Star Press, Fort Collins, CO.
4   Robinson SE and Fisher AG (1999) Functional and cognitive differences between cognitively well people and people with dementia. *British Journal of Occupational Therapy.* **62**(10): 466–71.
5   Pool J (1999) *The Pool Activity Level (PAL) Instrument*. Jessica Kingsley, London.
6   Thom KM and Blair SEC (1998) Risk in dementia: assessment and management – a literature review. *British Journal of Occupational Therapy.* **61**(10): 441–7.
7   Perrin T (2001) Don't despise the fluffy bunny: a reflection from practice. *British Journal of Occupational Therapy.* **64**(3): 129–34.
8   Perrin T and May H (2000) *Wellbeing in Dementia: an occupational approach for therapists and carers*. Churchill Livingstone, London.
9   Perrin T (1999) Occupational need in severe dementia: a descriptive study. *Journal of Advanced Nursing.* **25**(5): 934–41.

11

Social aspects of the assessment and treatment of dementia

Dorrie Ball and Nick Farrar

Developments in ways of viewing ageing

Dementia is predominantly a disorder of the very elderly population. It is claimed that at age 75, the prevalence of dementia is approximately 10% and this prevalence is doubled with every five years of increasing age.[1] Although there have been recent concerns in the discovery of 'new variant' Creutzfeldt–Jacob disease in patients aged 20–50 years, and there is increasing awareness that as people with learning disabilities are living longer they are particularly vulnerable to dementia, it is still the case that this disease is rare under the age of 65. However, whilst ageing appears to be the greatest risk factor in developing dementia, it must be stressed that dementia is not part of the normal ageing process.

In order to discuss the social aspects of the assessment and treatment of dementia, this chapter will initially explore the social context of older people, from theoretical and professional perspectives, with particular emphasis on the changes which have taken place in the last 10–15 years, so that issues of interventions and potential options in addressing dementia from a social perspective can be located in a current and realistic context. Other important issues to be considered include legislative and policy influences which have changed the role of social workers and other professionals, and placed increasing emphasis on the need for multidisciplinary working and the involvement of users and carers in the assessment process and the ongoing care.

Thompson suggests that working with older people in social care settings has in the past tended to be seen as routine and undemanding, requiring little expertise or training – a notion which he strongly challenges as a negative view, reflecting society's ageist and discriminatory attitude to older people.[2] This attitude can be manifested in many ways, such as direct oppression (e.g. abuse in its many forms) or more subtle forms, such as derogatory or patronising language, stereotypical humour in media presentations or jokes, or infantilisation – a process which sadly has often been observed in residential or other forms of institution (scheduled 'toileting' times, use of first names, etc.). A further significant element of this view of older people is the tendency to see ageing predominantly in medical terms and the ageing process as a period of degeneration rather than development, with inevitable links to illness and infirmity – the 'what do you expect at your age?' syndrome.

A decade ago, John Bond and colleagues suggested that there were a variety of theoretical approaches to addressing the study of ageing, emanating from biological, psychological and sociological perspectives which tended to focus on different aspects of the ageing process.[3] Biological perspectives expanded on the criteria suggested by Strehler[4] that ageing is universal, progressive, intrinsic to the organism and degenerative, and proposed theories of 'programmed' or 'unprogrammed' ageing. Psychological perspectives included experimental approaches which focused on measuring cognitive processes or developmental psychology, including the 'life-span' approach proposed by Eric Erikson.[5] Sociological perspectives included structuralist approaches, based on the belief that our social behaviour is the result of the organisation and structure of society. This led to explanations such as 'disengagement theory', which focused on the 'mutually beneficial withdrawal' of older people from society,[6] and its counterpart 'activity theory', whose emphasis was on maintaining continuity into older age.[7] From a political economy perspective there has been a focus on the 'structured dependency' of older people, which describes the dependent status resulting from restricted access to resources in society, particularly income following retirement.

Some of these theories may seem dated, but they are all approaches to the study of ageing and are not right or wrong, simply different – therefore resulting in different interventions. Bond *et al.* also suggested these approaches can be applied to dementia, thus clinical approaches would link to epidemiology/aetiology and hence to treatments; psychological approaches to developing cognitive tests and examining the sufferer's experience of the disease; and in contrast, sociological approaches would consider the social structure of society, with links to social class, etc., or focus on labelling (linked to diagnosis). This illustrates that there can be different disciplines, with different conceptual frameworks, which result in different ways of studying and interpreting the same phenomenon. However, these approaches may be complementary, each making a contribution to the understanding of dementia (ibid.). Thus they may be seen as contributing to a 'holistic' approach, a framework which is increasingly demanded by current policies and practice, such as multidisciplinary assessment.

The above theoretical approaches have presented ways of viewing ageing from a generalised perspective. In order to work with older people in an anti-oppressive and anti-discriminatory manner, it is essential to regard each older person as an individual with their own biography, which may be influenced by gender, race/ethnicity, class, sexual orientation, etc. It is also important to encompass changing life expectations over time, for example potential choices about retirement age, access to travel/holidays, life-long learning. Developments such as these may in time influence and change attitudes to older people, along with policy directives such as the National Service Framework for Older People, which sets national standards and defines service models for the care of older people, the first standard of which attempts to eliminate discrimination against older people in the provision of services.[8] Whilst this NSF addresses a broad range of policy and service issues, it also has a number of specific points which have significance for dementia care.

Developments in ways of working with dementia

The above theoretical explanations and changing perceptions of ageing have been reflected in the development of approaches to dementia over the last two decades. A leading exponent of new ideas in this field has been Tom Kitwood, whose personal experiences led to a growing interest and later a professional involvement in exploring ways of understanding and working with dementia.[9] Kitwood's ideas presented, initially rather tentatively, a challenge to the medical model which framed dementia as an 'organic mental disorder' or what he termed the 'standard paradigm'. His deepening involvement in enhancing the well-being and quality of care for dementia sufferers placed emphasis on authentic contact and communication, with a focus on 'person-centred care' and supporting family carers. A new method for evaluating the quality of care in formal settings was developed, termed 'dementia care mapping', which attempted to recognise the standpoint of the person with dementia, with consequent capacity to improve the caring process for both service users and carers.

Kitwood was not alone in promoting challenges to the biomedical theories of understanding dementia and the last decade has seen a proliferation of texts developing new approaches to care for people with dementia. It must, however, be pointed out that these innovative approaches have developed in a social and economic climate where there has been a major concern not only about the increasing number of people diagnosed as having dementia, but about the number of older people *per se*, whose increasing health and social care needs are perceived to be a 'burden' on welfare resources.

Many of the recent approaches have expanded on Kitwood's ideas of personhood and communication in dementia care, but there has also been a focus on the quality of care settings and the care environment, the development of a wide range of approaches to practice in this field, an emphasis on working with informal carers and the changes which the new policy context of the NHS and Community Care Act 1990 have effected in this field.[10] Concerns emanating in the mid-1980s about the disproportionate amount of funding and publicity for neurobiological research into dementia compared with research into care-giving perspectives resulted in an integrated multidisciplinary overview of the strategies and techniques available for use in caring for people with dementia,[11] followed by a further review of developments some five years later.[12] Both volumes attempted to address the wide range of models and theories which could be applied to dementia, as well as a range of potential interventions in care facilities, in the community and for the family, including the effects of culture, a range of psychosocial interventions and ways of supporting care-givers.

One entertaining and illuminating text, which emerged from a practical experiment to find the best way of intervening in the lives of people with dementia, resulted in a critique of the present state of theoretical and professional approaches. Its headings of 'Beyond the Biomedical Paradigm', 'Psychological and Linguistic Models', through 'Disease', and 'Diagnosis' to 'The Social

Construction of Dementia' tell their own story.[13] Other authors have argued that communication is at the heart of all approaches to dementia care, and have stressed the importance of developing new ways of communicating with and listening to people with dementia, in order to include their views in the designing and delivering of care.[14–16]

Within the social work field, Mary Marshall, a leading authority on working with older people, has claimed that working with people with dementia and their carers presents a range of exciting possibilities, which can include interventions from family therapy, creative use of the past, groupwork, etc.[17] Tibbs,[18] writing on social work and dementia, acknowledges Kitwood and others as innovators in developing holistic models of dementia, but notes that:

> The NHS and Community Care Act (1990) places social work on the purchaser side of the purchaser/provider equation, thus isolating them from the provider side growing body of knowledge.
>
> (p. 17)

It is suggested that there are a number of points when social workers may encounter people with dementia which combine some particular events connected to medical approaches (the time of diagnosis or admission to hospital) with life events, such as loss of particular memory skills or times when carers cannot cope and respite care is necessary (ibid., pp. 20–37). Tibbs reiterates many points of good practice such as the need for continuity of care and the need to support carers and be sensitive to carer stress. Especially important are specialist training, flexibility, accessible information and services, and the need for multi-disciplinary teams with psychologists (ibid., pp. 152). To deliver all of these very important practice developments, investment is needed.

Developments in care management and community care over the last ten years

Community care has a long history, but arguably the most dramatic changes in this country have come about over the last ten years, driven partly by the need to contain care costs of a population with a rising number of older people.

The NHS and Community Care Act 1990[19] ushered in a period of intense government activity, which continues in reshaping the delivery of social and healthcare.

These developments fall short of a complete 'joining up' of health and social care, but attempt to address issues in particular parts of the system in parallel and at the same time. One major focus is 'the user's view' – involving users and carers in planning and providing services to attempt to make the system 'a seamless service'. Another is separating assessment of need from provision of services to meet that need, which provides a 'gatekeeping' process of resources as well as targeting those who have the greatest need. Yet another focus is joint planning and joint target setting.[20]

Together these changes form part of an ongoing attempt to drive health and social care provision together, whilst keeping the essential differences between health and social care intact (healthcare being free at the point of delivery whilst social care is charged for) (ibid).

Two of the most recent national policy developments include Fair Access to Care Services (FACS),[21] which provides councils with an eligibility framework for delivery of adult social care services in each local area (i.e. who will get a service and who will not, based on a national set of needs-based criteria) and which has been introduced in 2003. In addition, the Single Assessment Process (SAP) described in the NSF for Older People sets out to co-ordinate the assessment process for older people right across the health and social care spectrum, with the intention of avoiding duplication, and to enhance information-sharing between professionals, and is due to be implemented in 2004.

Both of these will have significant implications for professionals and users alike. All of the above focus on user involvement in the whole system, empowering the service user and setting national standards and targets. They have potential advantages in that the standards and targets are public, and professionals and managers can be held to account for their delivery. In contradistinction, they can be seen as a strait-jacket for professional freedom. Getting the balance right is one of the biggest challenges to be faced in this environment. Risk as an essential part of health and social care has also been driven up the agenda for many reasons over the last ten years. What we must be aware of is that risk awareness does not become part of our plans to the detriment of appropriate risk taking.

What does this mean for people with dementia?

The Audit Commission's report 'Forget Me Not'[22] described the pattern of mental health services for older people in England and some of the recognised gaps, based on the current patterns of care delivery. These included more GP support and specialist training, the strengthening of specialist teams in half the areas, better comprehensive assessment facilities in day hospitals and more availability of appropriate respite care. In its update on the report in 2002, the Commission noted the close correlation between specialist services provided, teamwork and planning services. Where planning was good, services were seen to be good, and vice versa. What the report also noted, however, was that there was a wide range of performance, and it proposed that the introduction of the NSF for Older People should provide new impetus for all agencies to improve their services to the standards of the best practice.[23]

Thus we find that despite the changes so far made, where one lives still dictates the quality of care one gets. Structural changes cannot deliver changes of themselves. Much will depend on professional attitudes to these changes as to whether they have a significant impact on the way in which people are cared for. What we can say is that the stated intention is to change things for the better, and that the potential for more integrated assessment and provision of care is there.

The role of carers

There have been several legislative and policy developments in recent years which have relevance for carers of people with dementia. The Carers (Recognition and Services) Act 1995 was the first piece of legislation to formally recognise the role of carers. It ushered in the right of carers, who are providing substantial amounts of care on a regular basis, to have a separate assessment of their needs and ability to care, which local authorities are required to take into account when making decisions about providing services. However, research has suggested that separate carer assessments are not a standard feature of care management practice, and carers' access to services appears to be patchy.[24] Findings suggested that care managers' insight and understanding of the legislation were limited, there was a lack of clear policy at local level, and little specific training in relation to roles and responsibilities towards carers. Additionally, carers' knowledge of their rights to assessment was limited. Indeed, the study showed that 88% of carers were not informed of the Carers Act when the person with dementia was assessed and none were offered a separate assessment of their needs (ibid., p. 153).

Recognition of some of these limitations led to the National Carers Project in 1998, which resulted in the Carers' National Strategy.[25] This strategy placed emphasis on providing support to carers at key points in the caring process, and helping in the development of relevant skills. An important element of the strategy was the notion of giving carers the choice as to whether to care or not. However, achieving these apparently positive aims may not have been realistic, as most agencies tend to see carers as a resource and therefore attempt to maintain them in their role as far as possible.[26] It is suggested that there is a need to reach beyond the focus on the stress, burdens and physical aspects of caring, which much research has tended to address, to understand the multidimensional and dynamic nature of family care. This could point to a more holistic model of assessing carers' needs, rather than viewing them as a resource to be supplemented with additional services or to be superseded when caring has to cease. A model which proposes 'carers as experts' could offer an empowering approach which recognises not only the difficulties but the satisfactions and rewards of caring, and which gives equal prominence to the skills, abilities and expertise of carers as to the instrumental services such as respite care and housing support (ibid.).

The Carers and Disabled Children Act 2000 further developed the rights described in the 1995 Act by giving local authorities power to provide services directly to carers, even if the cared-for person did not wish for an assessment. This could include giving vouchers to the carer or user for short breaks, or providing direct payments to carers in lieu of services.

The Government has also provided some additional money for carers as part of its modernisation of social services initiative. A specific grant to social services departments – the Carers' Grant – was introduced in 1999 with a focus on the provision of breaks for carers, or services when carers cannot take advantage of a break. It has increased annually, and has been continued into 2003/4. The amount of the grant, in comparison to the actual costs of informal care, is small. Attempts to quantify the costs of informal care have met with difficulties as the relationship between measuring costs and key aspects of informal care is extremely complex, involving factors such as stress on carers, predictors of breakdown of caring networks and the effects of service interventions.[27] However, it can be assumed that if carers were to withdraw their support, the cost to the State would be colossal. A further point of relevance is that many people in relationships providing caring functions do not describe themselves as 'carers', rather regarding this as part of the close relationship or familial duty, which may particularly be the case with older carers or spouses. Additionally, it has been suggested that there is a pervasive assumption that women possess 'natural caring capacities' and will be available to care. As the largest proportion of informal (and formal) carers are women, caring predominantly for older women, this may reflect negatively on the perception of care arrangements for older people by compounding the negative stereotypes previously referred to.[28]

What difference will this make to people with dementia?

A national focus on supporting carers is of itself sensible, and necessary. As we have noted, the amount of informal care that takes place is of huge value, and society at large and the health and social care system rely very heavily on the goodwill of informal carers. A focus on carers is also very desirable from the point of view of individual service users and carers. However, studies show that caring for someone with dementia has particular challenges and stresses. Heron[29] has suggested that carers of people with mental health problems have traditionally been seen as a separate group of carers, with a distinct identity, even prior to the current interest in carers. Whilst carers in this group may benefit from generic support, specific needs may include information about the nature and progression of the illness, access to emergency services or short-term intensive interventions in the event of crises. Focusing resources on supporting people in these situations would clearly be of benefit to individual users and carers, and also of value to society at large.

The implications for interventions in the social aspects of dementia care

We have seen that there is now a much wider range of accepted views on dementia than there was ten years ago, which give us some basis for a more positive view on what can be achieved. The models of 'personhood' and the work on communication with people with dementia show what is possible, along with other new understanding about environment, illness, the person and their interaction with carers. We know that people with dementia can have valued lives, and that there is much that can be done to support this. In contradistinction, we can see from the Audit Commission analysis that there is much variation in services across the country, and that there is a strong correlation between planning, teamwork and good delivery. This means making sure that proper multidisciplinary planning and service delivery is made to work across the board – a challenge to the professions indeed.

So far, so good. If, however, we contrast that scenario with the current wider development of primary care trusts, and the stresses on them and on their staff to deliver many different targets, we come up with a mixed picture of possibilities, challenges and constraints. To advocate for people with dementia still is a necessary and tough task. The new possibilities raised by prescription of memory-supporting drugs (and advocated by the National Institute for Clinical Excellence) add to this picture another tantalising possibility with its concomitant debates about costs, expertise and 'who is in charge'. Even with the successful use of these drugs, however, there will still be people with dementia who need care.

In relation to the challenges to social care professionals, much of the above parallels the development of good practice in community care, which has been the emphasis since the implementation of the NHS and Community Care Act 1990. Key elements include a holistic approach to assessment, multidisciplinary teamwork (incorporating the movements towards merging health and social care introduced by many of the current government's policies), the development of service provision which addresses race equality strategies, and issues of partnership, participation and empowerment which infiltrate all of the above processes.

In relation to people with dementia, assessment and service provision would normally take place within the context of a multidisciplinary community mental health team. The advantages of this service context are that service users and carers receive a dedicated service, rationalised and co-ordinated service provision and specialised professional staff. The disadvantages (as in any multidisciplinary team) are that different professional and organisational cultures, interests and priorities can impede the assessment and service delivery process.[30] The challenge within this scenario is to achieve a balance between the social and medical models of dementia care.

A core theme of the assessment and care planning process is the emphasis on a needs-led approach – identifying individual needs and attempting to meet these needs, rather than slotting people into existing resources. Care management for people with dementia is not without its difficulties, such as balancing self-determination of the user with allowing acceptable levels of risk, and ensuring that the voice of the user is heard where articulation of their needs may be limited and the voice of the carer may seem to dominate. Much has been written in recent years to encourage the participation and empowerment of people with dementia, such as Barnett's inspiring text which addresses innovative ways of 'including the person with dementia in designing and delivering care' by learning to listen to the words that are said and reading the behaviour that we see.[31]

On a similar theme, Killick and Allan argue that communication is at the heart of all approaches to dementia care, and that maintaining positive developments in this sphere is the key to enhancing practice.[16] Several important principles arise from these proposals: firstly, the need for continuity of care, which may be difficult to achieve in organisational contexts of shift working, and staff movements and absences. Secondly, a very problematic issue is often the lack of time – one of the severe resource constraints – due to high workloads and low staff to user ratios versus the increased amount of time needed to communicate effectively with people with dementia. Thirdly, in order to develop new person-centred approaches, staff need to acquire specialist knowledge and skills. Trainers in one local social services department have developed an excellent range of training materials, incorporating modular packages addressing strategies and approaches reflecting the latest developments in dementia care, but maintain that the time available for training and the time staff can spend with clients are both extremely limited.[32]

Most developments in dementia care have focused on white ethnocentric approaches, and there has been limited research into the needs of ethnic minority communities in this respect. A study by Boneham et al. of Black British, Afro-Caribbean and Chinese older people diagnosed as suffering from dementia or depression suggested a low level of service despite considerable unmet need, due to communication difficulties, lack of knowledge of services or their inappropriateness culturally.[33] A later study by Adamson of African/Caribbean and South Asian families pointed to a lack of awareness of the condition of dementia and the need for appropriate information.[34] Both studies indicated that all the themes addressed in this chapter are exacerbated by cultural factors.

Although the emphasis of community care on maintaining older people in their own homes wherever possible applies equally to people suffering with dementia, it must be acknowledged that for some people this may not be possible, and a range of alternatives to home must be considered. Although there has been no coherent joint approach between housing policy and the broader context of health and social care policies, the importance of housing is paramount in providing quality in care settings. The report of the Royal Commission 'With Respect to Old Age: long-term care – rights and responsibilities'[35] provides a useful starting point for any analysis of possible models of supporting people in their own homes or in other settings. Within the report, the commissioners explore aspects such as intensive home support, co-resident care, very sheltered housing and assistive technology. The Report also notes: 'Dementia, more than physical incapacity, can present both family members and services with particular difficulties and extreme demands.'

Earlier government research had undertaken investigation of services for older people with dementia in the community by carrying out inspections of several local authorities.[36] Included in the main findings were the fact that the best practice appeared to occur where there were good collaborative arrangements between social services and NHS staff, particularly in relation to assessment, care management and service delivery, and that the commitment, knowledge and skills of many practitioner staff were high, though the need for training in specialist skills was vital. It was also noted that some areas of innovative practice were beginning to address a needs-led approach rather than rely on traditional services.

A concluding comment must be that the challenges and new directions for social care professionals working in the field of dementia care, in the current contexts of multidisciplinary policy and practice and organisational and financial constraints, must incorporate flexibility of approach and a wide range of perspectives in order to achieve good practice.

Key points

- There are many ways of viewing ageing – sociological, physical, psychological and biological – which have influenced views of dementia.
- There has been a dramatic development in new ways of thinking about dementia over the last 20 years. These new ways focus on positive person-centred care rather than a medical model.
- The many recent developments in community care have not necessarily addressed the needs of people with dementia.
- Services for people with dementia remain patchy, some very good, some poor.
- We still place a great degree of reliance on informal carers.
- The challenge is to use the new knowledge and the new ways of working in practice, with emphasis on interdisciplinary working, and placing the user at the centre of care. This means considerable work to break down professional barriers.

References

1 McKeith I and Fairburn A (2001) Biomedical and clinical perspectives. In: C Cantley (ed.) *A Handbook of Dementia Care*. Open University Press, Buckingham.
2 Thompson N (1995) *Age and Dignity: working with older people*. Arena/ Ashgate Publishing Ltd, Aldershot.
3 Bond J, Coleman P and Peace S (1993) *Ageing in Society: an introduction to social gerontology* (2e). Sage Publications, London.
4 Strehler BL (1962) *Time, Cells and Ageing*. Academic Press, London.
5 Erikson E (1950, 1965) cited in Bond J, Coleman P and Peace S (eds) (1993) *Ageing in Society: an introduction to social gerontology* (2e). Sage Publications, London.
6 Cumming E and Henry W (1961) *Growing Old: the process of disengagement*. Basic Books, New York.
7 Havinghurst RJ (1963) quoted in Bond J, Coleman P and Peace S (1993) (op.cit.) p. 32.
8 Department of Health (2001) *National Service Framework for Older People*. DoH, London.
9 Kitwood T (1997) *Dementia Reconsidered: the person comes first*. Open University Press, Buckingham.
10 Cantley C (2001) Understanding the policy context. In: C Cantley (ed.) *A Handbook of Dementia Care*. Open University Press, Buckingham.

11 Jones GMM and Miesen BML (eds) (1992) *Care-giving in Dementia: research and applications*. Routledge, London.

12 Miesen BML and Jones GMM (eds) (1997) *Care-giving in Dementia: Vol. 2*. Routledge, London.

13 Harding N and Palfrey C (1997) *The Social Construction of Dementia: confused professionals?* Jessica Kingsley, London.

14 Goldsmith M (1996) *Hearing the Voice of People with Dementia: opportunities and obstacles*. Jessica Kingsley, London.

15 Barnett E (2000) *Including the Person with Dementia in Designing and Delivering Care*. Jessica Kingsley, London.

16 Killick J and Allan K (2001) *Communication and the Care of People with Dementia*. Open University Press, Buckingham.

17 Marshall M (1993) New trends and dilemmas in working with people with dementia and their carers. In: A Chapman and M Marshall (eds) *Dementia: new skills for social workers*. Jessica Kingsley, London.

18 Tibbs MA (2001) *Social Work and Dementia: good practice and care management*. Jessica Kingsley, London.

19 *National Health Service and Community Care Act 1990*. HMSO, London.

20 Sharkey P (2000) *The Essentials of Community Care: a guide for practitioners*. Macmillan, Basingstoke.

21 Department of Health (2002) *Fair Access to Care Services*. HMSO, London.

22 Audit Commission (2000) *Forget Me Not: mental health services for older people*. Audit Commission, London.

23 Audit Commission Update (2002) *Forget Me Not 2002*. Audit Commission, London.

24 Seddon D and Robinson C (2001) Carers of older people with dementia: assessment and the Carers Act. *Health and Social Care in the Community*. 9(3): 151–8.

25 Department of Health (1999) *Caring about Carers: a national strategy for carers*. HMSO, London.

26 Nolan M and Keady J (2001) Working with carers. In: C Cantley (ed.) *A Handbook of Dementia Care*. Open University Press, Buckingham.

27 Netten A (1996) The costs of informal care. In: C Clark and I Lapsley (eds) *Planning and Costing Community Care*. Jessica Kingsley, London.

28 Orme J (2001) *Gender and Community Care: social work and social care perspectives*, pp. 99, 168. Palgrave, Basingstoke.

29 Heron C (1998) *Working with Carers*. Jessica Kingsley, London.

30 Millen J and Wallman-Durrant L (2001) Multidisciplinary partnership in a community mental health team. In: V White and J Harris (eds) *Developing Good Practice in Community Care: partnership and participation*. Jessica Kingsley, London.

31 Barnett E (2000) *Including the Person with Dementia in Designing and Delivering Care*. Jessica Kingsley, London.

32 Brook G and McDermott P (2000) *The Latest Developments in Dementia Care* and *A Modular Training Package (Modules One to Five)*. Training Department, Bradford Social Services Directorate.

33 Boneham MA, Williams KE, Copeland JRM *et al.* (1997) Elderly people from

ethnic minorities in Liverpool: mental illness, unmet need and barriers to service use. *Health and Social Care in the Community.* **5**(3): 173–80.

34 Adamson J (2001) Awareness and understanding of dementia in African/ Caribbean and South Asian families. *Health and Social Care in the Community.* **9**(6): 391–96.

35 Royal Commission on Long-term Care for Elderly People (1999) *With Respect to Old Age: long-term care – rights and responsibilities.* Research Vol. 2, p. 178. HMSO, London.

36 Department of Health/Social Services Inspectorate (1997) *At Home with Dementia: inspection of services for older people with dementia in the community.* HMSO, London.

12

The role of the memory clinic

Andrew M Ellis

Introduction

Initially a transatlantic invention of the mid-1970s, memory clinics have spread widely to offer outpatient diagnostic and treatment services for those suffering from memory difficulties. In Britain, the first such clinic was set up at University College Hospital, London in 1983[1] and by 1995, 20 active memory clinics were identifiable.[2] However, with the introduction of the acetylcholinesterase inhibitors to clinic practice since 1997, many new clinics have been developed to facilitate the treatment of patients with early and moderate Alzheimer's disease,[3] many of whom previously would not have been known to services.

Memory clinics have always served to offer a simple 'one-stop shop' approach to dementia, where patients could be comprehensively assessed, usually on a single visit, and informed later of their diagnosis and treatment options. However, their organisation has varied greatly, with the lead clinician usually being a consultant psychiatrist or psychologist, with a smaller number of clinics being run by a geriatrician or neurologist.[2] Most clinics take place in a hospital setting, with smaller numbers occurring in general practitioners' surgeries or in the community.

Staffing has similarly varied between clinics, but in most cases there is also specialist nursing and occupational therapy input. Psychologists have traditionally helped with formal neuropsychological testing, whilst a smaller number of clinics have involved other professionals, including speech therapists, physiotherapists and social workers who have assisted in providing the full assessment and counselling that such patients require. A growing number of clinics are also employing or allowing access to support workers from the Alzheimer's Society, for example, to provide additional care and counselling for patients and their carers.

Since the introduction of the new anti-dementia drugs, there has been a subtle change in role for many clinics. Whilst the focus had been on assessment and diagnosis of patients with dementia, with only limited pharmaceutical research, the availability of licensed treatments for Alzheimer's disease has given the memory clinics an additional role in the initiation and monitoring of treatment with these medications.

This chapter will concentrate on the many roles of the memory clinic in the assessment, diagnosis and treatment of people with suspected dementia, particularly focusing on practical issues in the setting up and running of such clinics.

Referrals

One of the initial issues that any memory clinic must address is the referral procedure and pathway. Deciding who can refer will determine the clinic population characteristics and will influence the proportions of clients who are subsequently diagnosed as having dementia. Previous studies have shown that if self-referrals are accepted then the prevalence rate of dementia will be 6%, whilst if referrals are accepted only through GPs, this rises to between 40–66% of patients seen.[4,5] These figures compare to community studies that show dementia prevalence rates between 0.5% and 16.3% for mild disease and 1.1% and 7.4% for moderate to severe illness.[6]

There may be specific reasons why a clinic would wish to take more self-referrals, and thus a lower prevalence rate of dementia at referral. Several centres are seeking to look at whether we can predict who will develop dementia, and there is some evidence that there is a higher rate of incident dementia in this population. Research could then assess whether specific treatments can delay the progression of early memory impairments into clinical dementia syndromes.

Treatment-focused clinics would, however, wish to increase the percentage of referred patients that might be suitable for medication, and one logical approach to this is to look at the production of a referral protocol defining who should be referred to the clinic. The Chester Memory Clinic has produced guidelines for its referrers (see Box 12.1) and these have been successfully used to ensure that a high proportion of referrals are suitable for treatment. Referral guidelines can also include advice on treatment for depression and delirium, and appropriate investigations that may aid diagnosis at an initial memory clinic appointment.

What about the remaining referrals?

Given the figures above, it is apparent that not all those who are referred to memory clinics will be diagnosed as suffering from a dementia. Whilst depression is the commonest other diagnosis, occurring in 6.5% of patients referred to a memory clinic run by a psychiatric team, 16.5% of referrals were felt to be 'well' with no formal diagnosis.[5] The same survey found a smaller number of patients where medical diagnoses were made (including hypothyroidism and Parkinson's disease), and a small proportion of referrals where no diagnosis could be made at the time of referral and retesting was advised.

Recently, a number of diagnoses have been proposed to classify these older people with poor memory, including age-associated memory impairment, benign

Box 12.1   The Chester Specialist Memory Clinic referral guidelines

Suggested guidelines for GP referral

Initially:
dementia should be considered if there is a loss of memory or skills in anyone for whom there is no other obvious cause.

There is a need to rule out:
- depression – the patient may be withdrawn, apathetic or indifferent to the assessment. Consider a trial of treatment for three months with a selective serotonin re-uptake inhibitor (SSRI) before referral.
- delirium – usually an acute history and quick deterioration. Characteristically has fluctuating level of consciousness: may be hallucinations and intense fearfulness.
- other causes, such as current drug treatment, including withdrawal or intoxication.

Initial assessment should include:
- history:
    - onset and course of cognitive impairment
    - degree of functional incapacity
    - current support from family, friends and statutory services.
- investigations:
    - full blood count
    - thyroid function tests
    - urea and electrolytes, liver function tests and calcium
    - urinalysis
    - ECG
    - chest X-ray (if clinically indicated).

Treatment will *not* be appropriate for:
- severe Alzheimer's disease (consider using Mini-Mental State Examination <12 as cut-off)
- patient unlikely to comply with medication.

Refer to specialist service:
when investigations rule out other obvious causes of cognitive problems. Please send results with referral to avoid duplication or delay.

Please also investigate support for patients and carers. Check to see if sources of further help are required (e.g. Alzheimer's Disease Society, social services).

senescence forgetfulness and ageing-associated cognitive decline. Although the status and validity of such diagnoses are unclear, current research indicates that while the majority of patients who receive such diagnoses do not go on to develop dementia, a small minority will, and that this occurs at a slightly higher rate than in the general population.[7]

The assessment process

Although clinics use different assessment protocols and methods, patients referred to memory clinics are then subject to a comprehensive programme of evaluation in order to establish whether or not a dementia is present, and to define the nature of that illness. Potentially treatable conditions such as depression or delirium need to be eliminated and treated, and reversible causes for dementias sought.

As with all psychiatric evaluations, the cornerstone of diagnosis remains that of a comprehensive psychiatric history and examination, though blood tests, appropriate radiological investigations and neuropsychological testing have considerable contributions to make.

Psychiatric history

A full history about the nature, severity and progress of the memory and other problems often requires other sources than the patient themselves who may have limited understanding or recall of their difficulties. A spouse or close family member is often the best informant and it may be necessary to interview them and the patient separately, particularly if they are anxious about divulging information about the patient in their presence. Great sensitivity is needed, and it may be necessary to supplement the information obtained by referral to the GP and hospital notes to gain a full medical history.

The principal aim of this history is to establish the pattern of difficulties and their development, and to look for symptoms and signs that point towards a diagnosis of dementia, and which may distinguish between the types of dementia. It is especially important to ask for symptoms of depression, which may be a cause for memory difficulties and is eminently treatable.

The history should also examine prescribed and non-prescribed drug use, looking for medication that may add to confusional states (for example, the anticholinergic effects of medication used for urinary incontinence or tricyclic antidepressants). Visual, hearing and language impairments, which may complicate neuropsychological examination, should be noted, as should the patient's educational and occupational history which gives an idea of pre-morbid attainments.

In view of the complexity of the information required, some clinics choose to use a standardised interview schedule to cover all the relevant points, often combining this with a scheme to establish diagnoses according to accepted international criteria.

Physical examination

This is important to exclude potentially treatable causes for the memory difficulties and to evaluate any co-morbid physical conditions. Reversible dementias are unfortunately rare, and occur only in around 1% of memory clinic referrals,[8] but physical conditions that may contribute to the cognitive problems are found in approximately 60% of patients seen.[9]

Blood tests

As there is no current diagnostic blood test for dementia, the focus of these investigations is to identify conditions that might themselves account for or compound memory problems. Routine screening should include full blood count to check for anaemia or infection, serum electrolytes to look for metabolic disease and thyroid function tests particularly to exclude hypothyroidism. If indicated, either on clinical history or the results of the full blood count, vitamin B_{12} and folate levels help rule out deficiency, and a serological test may help screen for neurosyphilis. Research clinics may also take further blood for genetic screening (for APOE status for example), but these tests have little current clinical utility.

Radiology

Most centres will have access to the structural imaging methods of CT and MRI scans. The main purpose of such scans is to exclude intracranial causes for the patient's symptoms (including tumours, abscesses, normal pressure hydrocephalus, infarcts, subdural haematomas and haemorrhages). Although MRI scans would often be the investigation of choice, because of their increased resolution and the ability to examine the brain in any plane, CT scans are often more practical as the procedure is quicker and less stressful for the patient. Functional imaging is less common at present with single photon emission computed tomography (SPECT) available at some centres and principally being used in research.[10]

Neuropsychological testing

Neuropsychological testing involves specialist skills and much effort on behalf of the patient and so careful consideration must be given to its purpose in assessing patients in the memory clinic.[11] Although designed to gain information about the specific deficits in cognitive functioning shown by patients, it can also help with diagnosis, particularly in patients with mild impairment, high pre-morbid intellectual ability or an unusual combination of symptoms. In such patients, testing to assess their previous intellectual ability may confirm that there has been deterioration, suggesting the presence of illness in someone who still scores well on other measures.

With increased emphasis on showing benefits of treatments, testing can also help to measure change by quantifying changes seen before and after medication.

Rating scales

Whilst a large number of rating scales are available to help assess those attending memory clinics,[12] it is important to make sure that these scales are appropriately used. Scales may need to be administered to patients, or an informant, or based on the observations of the rater. Some scales require specific training, whilst many others can be performed by any competent clinician. For patients with memory problems, ratings scales are available to assess:

- global severity and change

- degree of cognitive impairment

- behavioural and psychological symptoms

- abilities to perform the normal activities of daily living.

Depression rating scales are widely used as part of the screening process for both clients and carers. These and scales designed to rate care-giver burden and quality of life are often used to measure the effects of psychosocial interventions.

Global scales

Widely used in drug research trials, scales such as the Clinical Dementia Rating (A) and Clinician's Global Impression of Change (B) and their variants are usually completed by a clinician after a comprehensive interview with the patient and carer. If administered separately they may require up to 40 minutes to complete, but they can often be completed on the basis of the normal interviews taking place in the clinic.

Cognitive assessments

The most widely used rating scale for memory problems is the Mini-Mental State Examination (C), which has been extensively used to aid the assessment of cognitive impairment and for which age-specific normal scores are available. This assessment cannot replace full neuropsychological testing, as it is weak on testing for frontal lobe pathology for example. It was also not designed to measure change and indeed its test–retest and inter-rater reliabilities have been shown to be inadequate to detect the small changes in cognition expected with the currently available drug treatments for dementia.[13] Research trials of medication have therefore used the cognitive section of the Alzheimer's Disease Assessment Scale (ADAS-COG) (D). This must be administered by a trained interviewer and takes approximately 45 minutes, comprehensively testing 11 domains of cognitive function.

Many medical wards still use the Abbreviated Mental Test Score (E), a ten-item test that is helpful in screening for suspected cognitive impairment. Like the MMSE, it is relatively easy to administer, though recently newer screening tests such as the seven-minute neurocognitive screening battery (F) and the 6CIT (G) have been developed, claiming improved sensitivity and specificity in the detection of dementia.

Behavioural and psychological assessments

Both the Neuropsychiatric Inventory (NPI) (H) and Behave-AD (I) have been widely used in drug trials to examine behavioural and psychological symptoms of dementia. The NPI uses a number of screening questions to identify areas of difficulty before examining the frequency and severity of these symptoms. It takes about ten minutes to administer. The Behave-AD has sections concentrating on both the symptomatology and the severity of symptoms and takes 20 minutes.

Activities of daily living

From a practical point of view, how someone's memory affects their daily life is more important than the precise deficits in their memory. These activities of daily living have traditionally been assessed by occupational therapists, who can also suggest aids and helps to overcome some of the deficits found. When rating scales are used, an informant is usually necessary to obtain the information required.

The Bristol Activities of Daily Living (BADL) scale (J) was developed with carers to examine issues that carers rated as important in the daily living skills shown by patients with dementia, and measures 20 daily living skills. Thirty-three self-care activities are covered by the Interview for Deterioration in Daily Living Activities in Dementia (IDDD) (K), which also measures initiative and performance, whilst the Disability Assessment for Dementia (DAD) (L) is a newer observer-rated scale looking at basic activities of daily living.

Carer distress

Many carers experience considerable distress and even illness as a direct result of looking after someone with dementia, and whilst scales such as the Quality of Life in Alzheimer's Disease (QoL-AD) (M) have been specially developed, both depression rating scales and measures such as the General Health Questionnaire (GHQ) (N) have been used to detect psychiatric illness in them.

Depression scales

Depression rating scales are also used to detect depression in people with memory difficulties and include the semi-structured Hamilton Depression Rating Scale (HAM-D) (O) and the briefer Geriatric Depression Scale (GDS) (P).

Diagnosis

After the assessment process is complete, the multidisciplinary team must come to the conclusion as to whether a diagnosis can be confidently made at that time. If this is not possible, reassessment after a suitable delay may provide the additional evidence to support the presence or absence of a progressive dementia.

When diagnosis is possible, careful consideration must be given as to how the information is given to the patient and their carers. At present, only a minority of clinics routinely provide pre-test counselling, usually using models similar to those developed for HIV testing.[14] As the diagnosis of dementia has a major impact on the lifestyle and future plans of the individual and their carers, post-test counselling and support should also be available, both immediately and later when the impact of the diagnosis may be more apparent. In the past, professionals have often avoided these discussions as a consequence of the mistaken belief that the condition may stop the patient fully understanding the issues involved, though few now question the need to provide adequate information, support and advice to both patients and their carers. At the Chester Memory Clinic the employment of a family link worker jointly funded with the Alzheimer's Society has greatly enhanced this area of ongoing support to its clients.

Management

Although much of this section will concentrate on the practical aspects of drug treatment, an increasing number of clinics are also using other therapies to help people suffering from memory disorders. Programmes of memory training and other psychosocial interventions have their place, though are often only patchily available.[14] Attending a memory clinic in itself has been shown to improve the quality of life for carers,[15] and carer education and support groups add to this benefit, even delaying time to institutionalisation.[16]

Anti-dementia drugs

At present the principal class of anti-dementia medication is the anticholinesterase inhibitors (AChEIs). The original drug of this class, tacrine, was never widely used in Britain due to its liver toxicity, but there has been widespread but patchy uptake of the three newer medications, donepezil, rivastigmine and galantamine. No direct comparisons of these drugs are currently available, but there are some differences in the pharmacology of the three.[17] Whilst donepezil and galantamine are reversible inhibitors of acetylcholinesterase and are metabolised by the liver, rivastigmine is broken down by the acetylcholinesterase itself and is therefore described as 'pseudo-irreversible'. Donepezil has a significantly higher half-life of 72 hours, compared to between seven and eight hours for the other two drugs, allowing a once-daily rather than twice-daily dosage regimen. Their manufacturers have claimed that rivastigmine has an effect on a second enzyme, butyrl-cholinesterase, and galantamine has an action on nicotinic receptors, though the clinical effect of these actions is currently unknown. All three AChEIs are currently licensed for the treatment of mild and moderate Alzheimer's disease, though there is increased evidence of their effect in mixed (vascular and Alzheimer's disease) and Lewy body dementia.

There is limited evidence that vitamin E, an antioxidant, may have an effect on Alzheimer's disease, slowing down the development of dependency and delaying institutionalisation, and some evidence that nootropic agents such as gingko biloba extract may also be beneficial. Recently, a licence has been granted for the use of memantine, a blocker of N-methyl-D-asparate (NMDA) in moderate to severe dementia, though clinical experience of this drug is obviously limited.

Practical issues

Whilst the new anti-dementia drugs offer hope to patients and their carers, one of the most important tasks of the memory clinic is to manage the expectations of those taking these drugs. Those expecting a miracle cure will be disappointed, though in a progressively deteriorating illness even a decrease in the rate of decline may represent clinical benefit.

When these drugs were first introduced, research evidence of their clinical benefit was sparse and health authorities were wary of funding expensive treatments for a common condition. As a consequence patients tended to be given a time-limited trial of medication, after which benefit had to be shown to continue treatment. The National Institute for Clinicial Excellence[18] has recently reviewed the evidence for these drugs and published its recommendations, summarised in Box 12.2.[19]

Box 12.2   Summary of NICE guidelines on anti-dementia drug use

- All three drugs (donepezil, rivastigmine and galantamine) should be available in the NHS for those with mild and moderate Alzheimer's disease.
- The diagnosis must be made by a specialist according to standard diagnostic criteria.
- Cognition, global and behavioural functioning, and activities of daily living must be assessed before prescription, which is limited to secondary care. Cognitive function (MMSE) score must be >12.
- Compliance must be assured.

- Drugs should only be continued after assessment at two to four months showing:
  - improvement or no deterioration in MMSE score
  - evidence of global improvement on behavioural or functional assessment.
- Patients to be reviewed every six months and treatment continued only while MMSE score remains >12.
- Drug costs may be about £42m/year, which may be offset by delay into residential care.
- Specialised secondary care services need expanding, particularly memory clinics.

Current practice at the Chester Memory Clinic

After thorough assessment, patients with mild to moderate Alzheimer's disease may be suitable for a trial of an AChEI. The medical history should have identified any conditions that may preclude the drug use, such as active peptic ulceration, severe asthma and bradycardias where the heart rate is below 50 beats per minute. Similarly, the doctor should explore whether any additional illnesses need further treatment or whether any current treatments that could be adding to the difficulties can be safely changed.

Patients and their carers are then informed of the possible benefits and side-effects of the medications (principally gastrointestinal disturbance, insomnia, agitation and leg cramps), and of the fact that the medication is being prescribed for a trial period, after which benefit will be assessed. At the Chester Memory Clinic we have used a consent form for the treatment to ensure that this has taken place.

At this stage, compliance with medication is considered to determine whether the patient has someone who can ensure that the drugs are taken on a regular basis. The once-daily dosage of donepezil may be easier for those living alone, and compliance aids such as blister packs and Dossett boxes help if people are on several other medications. Finally, prescriptions are dispensed.

All three AChEIs are usually started at their lowest doses, with a programme of gradual titration to the maximum tolerated dose. A safety visit to the clinic at one month checks for problems with side-effects and then the patient attends for a fuller assessment at the end of the trial period.

Continuance of treatment after this visit is decided on the basis of the NICE guidelines. In addition to asking the patient and carer for their views on efficacy, a MMSE is performed, and repeat assessments of behavioural and psychological symptoms and activities of daily living made. The NICE guidelines suggested that medication should only be continued if there had been an improvement in MMSE score, or if there had been no change in MMSE score but evidence of improvement in daily living skills or behaviour.

If patients fail to show benefit then they are counselled and given advice about alternative treatments (including vitamin E and gingko biloba). Ongoing support is offered outside the clinic via the community mental health teams, who are informed of the decision to discontinue treatment at this time.

After the initial trial of treatment, patients continuing on medication are monitored by the clinic, with further assessments after every six months on the treatment.

One of the more controversial recommendations of NICE was that medication should not normally be continued in patients whose MMSE score had fallen below 12. Anecdotal reports of dramatic declines in patients where AChEIs are stopped are common, and as a consequence many clinics currently either ignore this recommendation or conduct a brief trial off medication in these patients. If decline does occur, it is usually rapid, and if the drug is restarted quickly, may be alleviated.

Research and audit

Before the widespread availability of drugs, many clinics were involved in research into treatments for dementia.[2] Whilst drug–placebo trials may no longer be ethical in Alzheimer's disease when licensed drugs are available, research is still needed into the effects of these drugs in other dementias and to compare these medications. Several practical questions remain unanswered, including whether combination therapies are beneficial and defining the place of switching from one drug to another. Predictors of drug response have yet to be identified and genetic studies may still provide vital evidence in this area.

Research continues to develop psychosocial interventions and evaluate their benefits, and ongoing audits of clinic practice can improve the quality of service that memory clinics offer.

Education and training

As specialists in the assessment of people presenting with memory difficulties, memory clinic professionals are well qualified to teach others about recognising dementia and raise awareness of these diseases amongst health professionals. Many opportunities exist for this, including during the formal pre-qualification training of each healthcare specialist as well as the programmes of continuing professional development required by each healthcare speciality.

Most primary care practices now have regular team meetings and usually welcome training on the detection of dementia in their patients. Comprehensive feedback to them about patients referred for assessment also teaches them about dementia, and difficult-to-diagnose patients discussed either by phone or in person improves working relationships with colleagues in primary care and adds to a joint understanding of the issues involved in the diagnosis of dementia. The primary care practitioner is often more aware of the family and social issues surrounding their patients and similarly can often enlighten memory clinic workers.

In addition, both local postgraduate education meetings and national conferences provide places where the operation of the local clinic can be publicised, teaching others about the comprehensive assessment of patients with dementia and helping to disseminate good clinical practice to other centres. Many memory clinics welcome enquiries from interested professionals and informal visits to other centres can highlight practical issues in running such clinics, particularly helpful to those about to set up a memory clinic service.

Setting up a memory clinic

As with any service development, it is important to define the role and purpose of a new memory clinic. There must be clear patterns of referral and good links with existing services. Box 12.3 shows some questions to consider before starting a clinic.[20]

Box 12.3   Some questions for a new memory clinic service

Why have a memory clinic?
- What is the core function of the proposed memory clinic?
- How will clients be referred to the service?
- What inclusion and exclusion criteria will operate?
- How will it improve the service already available to clients, carers, staff and referrers?
- Will it become the main or only access to dementia services?
- Will it offer diagnoses?
- Will it be a centre for dementia drug trial research?
- Will it replace other assessment services?

Ethical issues
- How will the client's consent to assessment and treatment be obtained?
- How will the decision be made about what to tell the client concerning the clinic's findings?
- Who will discuss the findings with the client and carer?
- How will the clinic deal with concerns about a client continuing to undertake activities that staff feel they are no longer able to do safely, for example driving?

Practical issues
- Who will work in the clinic?
- How will their tasks be allocated?
- What blood tests and physical investigations are required by the clinic?
- Who will perform these?
- Will a pre-clinic screening test be used?
- What tests will be used in the clinic?
- Will pre-test counselling be offered?
- Will post-test counselling be offered?
- What links will the clinic have with other health, social and voluntary sector services?
- How will the clinic be funded?

Increasingly, there is a need to develop a good business case to persuade others of the benefit of providing a memory clinic service. Further to the NICE guidelines,[18] there has been pressure on health authorities and trusts to fund the new drug treatments for dementia.[19] Memory clinics can be proposed as a way of ensuring that these treatments are targeted effectively and that their benefit is established for individuals, but care must be taken to make sure that an overstretched clinic with a long waiting list does not provide a 'back-door' rationing for these therapies. Memory clinics have also been supported by the Audit Commission 'Forget Me Not' report[21] as being valuable for their role in co-ordinating assessment and treatment for people with memory difficulties. The benefits for both clients and carers have been demonstrated, and carers and clients often become passionate advocates of the service.

It is difficult to predict demand for a new service, though a doubling of referrals by the third year of operation has been shown in one clinic.[22] This suggests a need to define the capacity of the clinic for new referrals and to agree with interested parties a procedure for regular funding reviews.

The future of memory clinics

Memory clinics are constantly changing. From the few diagnostic and drug-research clinics of the 1980s have come the many assessment and treatment clinics of today. The increasing demand for assessment and treatments is likely to continue as the general population ages and public knowledge of therapies increases. If the memory clinics are to carry on such a comprehensive service for drug therapies, either considerable resources will have to be found or alternative ways of monitoring developed. Clinics are starting to develop 'shared-care' protocols to monitor treatment with the patient's own GP, though these are still in their infancy. Clinics are also moving out of their central bases, and increasingly taking the assessments to their clients in their own homes, integrating more closely with existing community teams. Such 'virtual clinics' collate their results centrally for research purposes, often negating the need for special premises.

Memory clinics are also ideally placed to lead in the development of services for patients with early dementias. Before the availability of treatments, clinicians had largely ignored this group of patients, but they have considerable needs for help in adjusting to their diagnosis and making plans for their uncertain future.[23]

Such future developments are exciting, but will continue to provide several challenges to the ways that memory clinics currently function.

Key points

- Memory clinics have developed since the 1970s to provide a thorough assessment of people presenting with memory problems.
- Comprehensive assessment should be multidisciplinary and will always involve a thorough psychiatric history, physical examination, appropriate blood and radiological investigation, and neuropsychological testing.

- Rating scales must be used appropriately but can provide important information for assessment and monitoring of all interventions, both psychosocial and pharmaceutical.
- Consideration must be given to the psychological needs of patients and their carers; pre-screening and post-diagnosis counselling should be more widely available in memory clinics.
- The new anticholinesterase inhibitors have provided hope for patients and their carers. Current guidelines recommend a trial of treatment and continuation of these drugs only if benefit is proven.
- Memory clinics are well placed to lead in the development of services for people with early dementia, including psychosocial interventions.

References

1 van der Cammen TJM, Simpson JM, Fraser RM *et al.* (1987) The memory clinic: a new approach to the detection of dementia. *British Journal of Psychiatry.* **150**: 359–64.
2 Wright N and Lindesay J (1995) A survey of memory clinics in the British Isles. *International Journal of Geriatric Psychiatry.* **10**: 379–85.
3 Evans M, Ellis A, Watson D *et al.* (2000) Sustained cognitive improvement following treatment of Alzheimer's disease with donepezil. *International Journal of Geriatric Psychiatry.* **15**: 50–3.
4 Kelly CA, Harvey RJ, Nicholl CG *et al.* (1995) Specialist memory clinics: the experience at the Hammersmith Hospital. *Facts and Research in Gerontology.* **1**: 21–30.
5 Dennis M, Furness L, Lindesay J *et al.* (1998) Assessment of patients with memory problems using a nurse-administered instrument to detect early dementia and dementia subtypes. *International Journal of Geriatric Psychiatry.* **13**: 405–9.
6 Jorm AF, Korten AE and Henderson AS (1987) The prevalence of dementia: a quantitative integration of the literature. *Acta Psychiatrica Scandinavica.* **76**: 465–79.
7 O'Brien JT (1999) Age-associated memory impairment and related disorders. *Advances in Psychiatric Treatment.* **5**: 279–87.
8 Walstra GJ, Teunisse S, van Gool WA *et al.* (1997) Reversible dementia in elderly patients referred to a memory clinic. *Journal of Neurology.* **244**: 17–22.
9 Hogh P, Waldemar G, Knudsen GM *et al.* (1999) A multidisciplinary memory clinic in a neurological setting: diagnostic evaluation of 400 consecutive patients. *European Journal of Neurology.* **6**: 279–88.
10 O'Brien J and Barber B (2000) Neuroimaging in dementia and depression. *Advances in Psychiatric Treatment.* **6**: 109–19.
11 Morris RG, Worsley C and Matthews D (2000) Neuropsychological assessment in older people: old principles and new directions. *Advances in Psychiatric Treatment.* **6**: 356–61.

12 Burns A, Lawlor B and Craig S (1999) *Assessment Scales in Old Age Psychiatry.* Martin Dunitz, London.

13 Bowie P, Branton T and Holmes J (1999) Should the Mini-Mental State Examination be used to monitor dementia treatements? *Lancet.* **354**: 1527–8.

14 Royan L (2000) The memory clinic: current status and psychosocial interventions. *CPD Bulletin Old Age Psychiatry.* **2**(2): 37–9.

15 Logiudice D, Waltrowicz W, Brown K *et al.* (1999) Do memory clinics improve the quality of life of carers? a randomized pilot trial. *International Journal of Geriatric Psychiatry.* **14**: 626–32.

16 Brodaty H, Gresham M and Luscombe G (1997) The Prince Henry Hospital Dementia Care-givers' Training Programme. *International Journal of Geriatric Psychiatry.* **12**: 183–92.

17 Bullock R (2002) New drugs for Alzheimer's disease and other dementias. *British Journal of Psychiatry.* **180**: 135–9.

18 National Institute for Clinical Excellence (2001) *NICE Guidance on the Use of Donepezil, Rivastigmine, and Galantamine for the Treatment of Alzheimer's Disease.* Technology Appraisal Guidance No. 19. NICE, London.

19 O'Brien JT and Ballard CG (2001) Drugs for Alzheimer's disease. *British Medical Journal.* **323**: 123–4.

20 Sutton L (1998) Setting up a memory clinic. *Psychologists Special Interest Group in the Elderly (PSIGE) Newsletter.* **63**: 9–22.

21 Audit Commission (2000) *Forget Me Not: mental health services for older people.* Audit Commission, London.

22 Voss S, Bullock R and Rose C (2001) Don't forget. *Geriatric Medicine.* **31**(5): 51–3.

23 Moniz-Cook E and Woods RT (1997) The role of memory clinics and psychosocial intervention in the early stages of dementia. *International Journal of Geriatric Psychiatry.* **12**: 1143–5.

Further reading

Agency for Health Care Policy and Research (1996) *Clinical Practice Guideline No. 19: recognition and initial assessment of Alzheimer's disease and related dementias.* US Department of Health and Human Services, Rockville, MD.

Agency for Health Care Policy and Research (1996) *Quick Reference Guide for Clinicians No. 19: recognition and initial assessment of Alzheimer's disease and related dementias.* US Department of Health and Human Services, Rockville, MD.

Rating scales

A   CDR

Hughes CP, Berg L, Danziger WL *et al.* (1982) A new clinical scale for the staging of dementia. *British Journal of Psychiatry.* **140**: 566–72.

B   CGIC
Guy W (1976) Clinical global impressions. In: W Guy (ed.) *ECDEU Assessment Manual for Psychopharmacology*, pp. 218–22. Revised DHEW Pub. (ADM), National Institute for Mental Health, Rockville, MD.

C   MMSE
Folstein M, Folstein S and McHugh P (1975) Mini-Mental State: a practical method for grading the cognitive state of patients for the clinician. *Journal of Psychiatric Research*. **12**: 189–98.

D   ADAS-COG
Rosen W, Mohs R and Davis KL (1984) A new rating scale for Alzheimer's disease. *American Journal of Psychiatry*. **141**: 1356–64.

E   AMTS
Hodkinson H (1972) Evaluation of a mental test score for assessment of mental impairment in the elderly. *Age and Ageing*. **1**: 233–8.

F   **Seven-minute neurocognitive screening battery**
Solomon PR, Hirschoff A, Kelly B *et al.* (1998) A seven-minute neurocognitive screening battery highly sensitive to Alzheimer's disease. *Archives of Neurology*. **55**: 349–55.

G   **6CIT: Kingshill version**
Brooke P and Bullock R (1999) Validation of the six-item cognitive impairment test. *International Journal of Geriatric Psychiatry*. **14**: 936–40.

H   NPI
Cummings JL, Mega M, Gray K *et al.* (1994) The Neuropsychiatric Inventory: comprehensive assessment of psychopathology in dementia. *Neurology*. **44**: 2308–14.

I   **Behave-AD**
Reisberg B, Borenstein J, Salob SP *et al.* (1987) Behavioural symptoms in Alzheimer's disease: phenomenology and treatment. *Journal of Clinical Psychiatry*. **48** (suppl. 5): 9–15.

J   **BADL**
Bucks RS, Ashworth DI, Wilcock GK *et al.* (1996) Assessment of activities of daily living in dementia: development of the Bristol Activities of Daily Living scale. *Age and Ageing*. **25**: 113–20.

K   IDDD
Teunisse S, Derix MM and van Crevel H (1991) Assessing the severity of dementia. *Archives of Neurology*. **48**: 274–7.

L   DAD
Gelinas I, Gauthier L and McIntyre M (1999) Development of a functional measure for persons with Alzheimer's disease: the Disability Assessment for Dementia. *American Journal of Occupational Therapy*. **53**: 471–81.

M   QoL-AD
Logsdon RG, Gibbons IE, McCurry SM *et al.* (1999) Quality of life in Alzheimer's disease: patient and care-giver reports. *Journal of Mental Health and Ageing.* **5**: 1.

N   GHQ
Goldberg DP and Williams P (1998) *A User's Guide to the General Health Question-naire.* NFER-Nelson, Windsor.

O   HAM-D
Hamilton M (1960) A rating scale for depression. *Journal of Neurology, Neurosur-gery and Psychiatry.* **23**: 56–62.

P   GDS
Yesavage JA, Brink TL, Rose TL *et al.* (1983) Development and validation of a geriatric depression screening scale: a preliminary report. *Journal of Psychiatric Research.* **17**: 37-49.

13

Towards practical service delivery for younger people with dementia

Tony Dearden

Introduction

In recent years there has been a growing recognition that younger people with dementia and their carers can have very different needs to older people and that existing health and social care provision is very poorly adjusted to accommodate these differences. The historical division of health and social services, based upon the age of 65 years, has often resulted in patients, and carers, being marooned between general psychiatry, old age psychiatry and neurology.

Addressing the needs of early onset dementia sufferers, that is, those people with dementia who are under 65 years of age, and their families, presents a serious organisational challenge to all agencies. In addition, the early onset dementias are a very heterogeneous group of disorders with widely varying presentations, quite different cognitive and physical impairments as well as a wide range of psychiatric and behavioural features, which will challenge any clinical team. The aims of this chapter are to summarise the key issues, both clinical and organisational, as space does not allow for detailed discussion. However, it is the intention to indicate where improvements to clinical care should and can be made, based on published evidence and practical experience.

Differences?

The management of younger patients can present different problems because of their different social, economic and family circumstances. The ways in which the needs of younger people may differ from those over 65 include the following:

- Younger people are more likely to be in work at the time of diagnosis.
- Carers of younger people with dementia are likely to face different life conditions to carers of older people.
- Younger people are likely to be more active than older people, their physical strength may be greater and behaviour may be more problematic.

- Younger people are more likely to have dependent children and heavy financial commitments.

- They experience different emotional reactions. For both the person with dementia and their family, the diagnosis has a dramatic effect on future life plans and expectations.[1]

Genetic aspects and the issue of inheritance are of greater concern and more common. There is a higher prevalence of the 'rarer dementias' and clinicians need the awareness, knowledge and experience to work with the different needs presented by the whole range of dementias.

However, it is important to recognise that the 'age 65 cut-off' is biological nonsense and that people experience a continuum of physical, psychological and social changes. There are also a great many similarities between dementia in younger and older people, the key principles of good quality care are the same, and the knowledge and skills used in one area of practice can be transferred to another.

The experiences of people with early onset dementia and their families

There have been a number of local studies in different parts of the UK assessing the needs of younger people with dementia. A review of the literature reveals the main areas of concern to most, if not all, sufferers, carers and service providers to be:

Difficulties in assessing the numbers and levels of demand

Alternative methods of determining prevalence and incidence have produced widely varying figures. This has resulted in uncertainty, with service providers anxious that resources will be insufficient for the demand and commissioners reluctant to invest in the development of a service that might subsequently be underused. Fortunately there is now an adequate evidence base and a lot of practical experience from around the country that enables clinicians and managers to predict the numbers and quantify the likely service needs of a local population (see below).

Poor service articulation and co-ordination

The relatively low prevalence and incidence of early onset dementia means that there are often no clearly articulated pathways to appropriate diagnosis, assessment and aftercare existing for this client group. Referrals for diagnosis are made to a diverse range of health professionals, including neurologists, psychiatrists, psychologists and physicians. As a result, people frequently end up receiving either no care at all in the initial stages of dementia or widely differing packages of care. People with dementia and their carers can be left unsupported for some time after diagnosis, and only after a crisis point has been reached do support services become involved.

Problems with information and advice

Patients and carers frequently report that insufficient information is given at, and after, diagnosis regarding the nature of the illness and the availability of support services. Great sensitivity is needed to determine how much information people are ready to receive and when it is appropriate to give such information and advice. Carers and sufferers need information about the illness and its effects, financial and legal advice, information on available health, social and voluntary sector provision, and advice on coping with psychiatric and behavioural problems.

Inappropriate support services

Younger people with dementia are frequently reluctant to receive elderly services when they are provided because they feel that they do not belong in a setting where other users are usually very much older and less active than they are. Similarly, under-65 adult mental health services are usually intended for people with very different needs and are rarely able to provide the degree of supervision required by people with dementia, resulting in the danger of younger people being 'orphaned in a no man's land' between services.

The burden of coping

Early onset dementia is characterised by a high psychiatric and behavioural morbidity compared with late onset dementia.[2,3] These non-cognitive symptoms are particularly stressful to carers, and research has shown them to be even more strongly associated with care-giver burden than other very powerful influences such as the degree of impairment and the duration of dementia.[4,5] These very high levels of carer burden are thought in turn to lead to greater levels of service use.

How many?

As someone involved for some time in developing services for younger people with dementia, I have heard many clinicians express concerns that they would become overburdened by the number of patients (high) whilst at the same time listening to managers express concerns that they could not justify investment for the number of people involved (low). Therefore, the availability of reasonably accurate estimates of the frequency of early onset dementia, i.e. incidence and prevalence data, should help remove some of the uncertainty and anxiety for health service planners, managers and clinicians and encourage the development of needs-led and cost-effective services.

The different methodologies employed by researchers and clinicians in the various epidemiological and local needs assessment studies have produced in the literature a wide range in the rates of prevalence and incidence in any given population. However, the larger studies with good case definition and sampling methods do give very similar findings. What follows is not intended to be a scientific exposition of the complex epidemiological issues, but the headline information and evidence that should be useful to those developing services.

Research by Newens et al.,[6] investigating Alzheimer's disease only, reported a prevalence of 34.6 per 100 000 people between the ages of 45–64 years. This finding has been replicated by Harvey,[2] who reported a rate of 35 per 100 000 for the same age range. The same study also examined the rates of other causes of early onset dementia in two London boroughs and a summary of this population by type of dementia is shown in Figure 13.1.

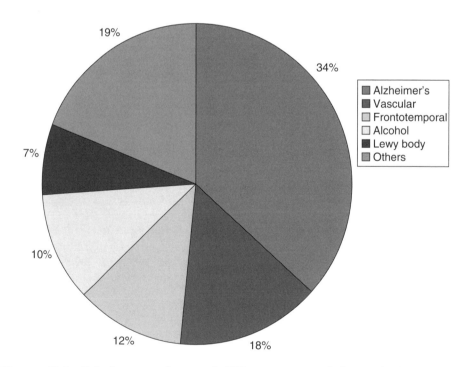

Figure 13.1 Relative prevalence of different types of dementia in younger people.

It can be seen that only one in three cases of early onset dementia is due to Alzheimer's disease, a significantly lower proportion than in later life. Many clinicians working in this field have found even lower rates than quoted for Lewy body dementia, a very common condition amongst 70 and 80-year-olds with dementia. In contrast, frontotemporal dementia accounts for one in seven cases of early onset dementia, although it appears to be underdiagnosed in clinical practice. Alcoholic dementia is a condition of the young and it can be seen that a much higher proportion of cases compared to older adults are due to other causes. The most common and important other causes include Huntington's disease, dementia in multiple sclerosis, corticobasal degeneration, connective tissue diseases, metabolic disorders, neurosyphilis, normal pressure hydrocephalus and prion diseases.

Given that the numbers of people with the non-Alzheimer's dementias are inevitably small, the frequency rates reported are less reliable and less consistent. However, the epidemiological study by Harvey[2] found the prevalence rate for all causes of dementia in 45–64 year-olds to be 98 per 100 000. This is compatible with other epidemiological work – therefore I recommend to planners as a 'good rule of thumb' to determine the number of cases in their local population, using the figure of 1 per 1000 in 45–64 year-olds.

Dementia is very rare before the age of 45 years with around 10% of early onset cases occurring before this age, mostly caused by rare and unusual diseases. Plotting the number of cases of dementia against age produces an exponential curve (see Figure 13.2), exemplified by the prevalence and incidence of Alzheimer's disease, which approximately doubles every five years from the age of 40 years onwards.

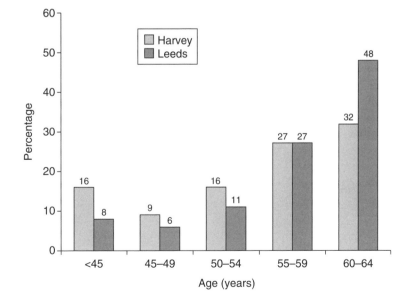

Figure 13.2   Distribution of dementia by age of onset.

Table 13.1   Abnormal genes identified in the dementias

	Gene	Chromosome
Alzheimer's disease	Amyloid precursor protein (mutations)	21
	Presenilin-1 (mutations)	14
	Presenilin-2 (mutations)	1
Creutzfeldt–Jacob disease	Prion protein: PRNP (mutations)	20
Frontotemporal dementia	Tau (mutations)	17
Huntington's disease	Huntington (CAG trinucleotide expansion)	4

Studies of risk factors in early onset dementia have investigated genetic and environmental factors. There is now a huge body of literature on the genetics and molecular pathology of Alzheimer's disease in particular. The abnormal genes identified in the dementias are summarised in Table 13.1.

Some authors have speculated that all cases of early onset Alzheimer's disease might be inherited as an autosomal dominant trait, not withstanding that many cases have no family history. A number of studies then attempted to determine the proportion of familial cases and to assess the relative risk of dementia in the relatives of probands. The most extensive survey, to date, of a population-based series of 101 familial and sporadic cases of early onset AD, applying modern molecular genetic techniques to screen for mutations, showed an overall prevalence for mutations of only 7%: 6% presenilin-1 and 1% presenilin-2 with no cases of APP mutations.[7] When only those with a clear family history were included in the analyses, the prevalence of mutations rose to 18%. These data suggest that the identified gene mutations for Alzheimer's disease are rare and account for less than one-fifth of cases with a family history.

Diagnosis and assessment

In practice, the experienced clinician can make a diagnosis in two ways. Both involve taking a history and informant history, with the aim of establishing the mode of onset, evolution, pattern and impact of any deficits, together with mental state examination, cognitive assessment, neuropsychological testing, physical examination, investigations and neuroimaging. The first method is 'pattern recognition'. That is, based on experience and knowledge of different disorders, do these symptoms and signs match any patient/syndrome I have previously seen? Do the different pieces of the jigsaw, history to neuroimaging, fit together into a meaningful whole? The second method is 'systematic analysis'. This is based on two fundamental facts: that cerebral diseases do not affect the brain uniformly, but preferentially affect certain brain regions and spare others, and that mental/psychological processes themselves are regionally organised and depend upon the functioning of specific brain regions. It follows, therefore, that the causative disease or pathology can be deduced after the precise neuropsychological deficits have been determined.

Four main groups of patients are seen: the worried-well, the psychiatrically ill (particularly depression), those with a degenerative dementia and a miscellaneous group (with focal brain pathologies, delirium, etc.). The first aim of identifying the worried-well is often made more complicated because the worry is generated by a positive family history. For a significant number, follow-up over time will be the only way of making absolutely sure that subtle complaints do not herald the onset of an organic syndrome.

The proportion of cases with a potentially reversible disorder will vary according to referral patterns. Numerous systemic disorders can potentially give rise to cognitive impairment, and so it is important to take a detailed past history to see if any candidates turn up. Of particular importance are markers of vasculitis such as rash, arthritis or renal disease and metabolic disorder, e.g autoimmune thyroid disease. The traditional infection related to cognitive impairment, syphilis, is now rare in the western world but still occurs occasionally. HIV and its complications, e.g. progressive multifocal leukoencephalopathy, is now the leading infectious cause of chronic cognitive impairment.

The most common treatable differential diagnosis of degenerative dementia is psychiatric illness, particularly depression. Symptoms of mood disturbance (anhedonia, pessimistic ruminations, suicidal ideas) and biological features of depression (anorexia, early morning waking, reduced libido) should be sought in all cases. It is important to note, however, that a significant number of those with organic brain disorders will exhibit concurrent psychiatric symptoms, particularly features of depression. Follow-up may be the only way of separating depression with cognitive symptoms from dementia with prominent affective symptoms.

For those who show evidence of organic impairment of cognition, the aim is to reach a specific diagnosis. A useful subclassification is into those with a relatively pure cognitive syndrome and those with associated neurological signs. The clinical patterns for the major degenerative dementias are summarised in Table 13.2.[8]

Difficulties in obtaining a diagnosis of dementia appear to be greater before the age of 65 years. Yet, an early diagnosis is important since it enables patient, family and carers to have a greater understanding of the illness and prognosis, and a better opportunity to attend to work and family responsibilities and to plan the management of the illness and for the future. Delayed diagnosis causes distress for patients and the families of people with dementia. An Australian study reported that the diagnostic process was considered problematic by 71% of carers, with 21% reporting misdiagnosis, the mean time to diagnosis was 3.4 years, and that the diagnosis was only made after patients had seen an average of 2.8 health service professionals.[9] Diagnosis is more easily missed when not suspected because of patient age, when symptoms are denied by patient, family and colleagues, when symptoms are misdiagnosed as due to functional disorders,[10] or when behavioural or personality changes are the first symptoms, as they are in certain dementia syndromes.

Table 13.2　Clinical patterns for the major degenerative dementias

	Memory	Language	Visuo-spatial	Attention	Frontal behavioural symptoms	Neurological signs
Alzheimer's disease	++++	++	++	++	+/−	−
Alzheimer's: biparietal variant	+/++	+	++++	++	+/−	−
Dementia with Lewy bodies	++	+	+++	+++	+/−	++
Frontotemporal dementia						− (unless associated with MND)
Semantic dementia	+	++++	+/-	+	++	
Frontal variant	+	+	+/-	++	++++	
Progressive aphasia	+/-	++++	+/-	+	+	
Corticobasal degeneration	+	+	+++	++	++	+++
Progressive supranuclear palsy	+	+	+	+++	++	+++
Huntington's disease	+	+	+	+++	++	+++

MND = motor neurone disease

Every patient then requires a comprehensive assessment of needs and risks in order to produce an individual care plan tailored to specific needs to enhance quality of life. This should include determining functional ability and impact upon daily living as well as the presence of particular problems, such as driving safety and risk, which applies to a much greater proportion of patients than in a service for older people. The needs assessment must also identify action required for financial support and benefits, activities, personal care, hygiene, feeding and housing. Clinical staff must also assess eligibility for treatment with cholinesterase inhibitors, or the use of other psychiatric medications, e.g. antipsychotics, and the appropriateness of behavioural and psychotherapeutic management. Families and carers also need to be interviewed with a particular reference to assessment of their mental and physical health and coping styles.

Information, care and support

It can be difficult for doctors to know how much information to give to the person with dementia and their family. Professionals are often fearful of giving the diagnosis of dementia: 'it will be too upsetting' or 'there is no treatment'. The danger is that very limited information or false reassurance can make caring and planning even more stressful.

There is no doubt that the person with dementia has 'the right to know'. In practice, most people with early onset dementia, in the early stages of the disease, know there is something wrong. The commonest fears are that they are going mad, or have a brain tumour. If giving the diagnosis is handled sensitively and positively, with the assurance of long-term support and help, then it is rarely as devastating as the person giving it imagines it will be, and people are relieved to know the diagnosis. If the diagnosis is made early enough and shared, the person with dementia can play a very active part in the planning of their future care.

Sometimes people do not wish to know the name of their illness, and sometimes they deny it when it is given. In these situations, it is accepted that someone has a right not to have the name forced on them. It is important to explain the cause of the memory impairment and other cognitive, emotional and personality changes occurring as a consequence of brain changes. Often the knowledge that repetitive questioning or conversation, emotional changes, lack of care and concern, loss of skills, poor personal hygiene and poor recent memory are due to a disease process, and not wilful 'awkwardness', is in many ways a relief.

The person giving the diagnosis should emphasise the positive aspects of what can be done to help the person with dementia and others, as well as giving an account of the specific illness and the course it is likely to take. The course and rate of progression of dementia varies dramatically between different diseases. Older patients with Alzheimer's disease may live for up to 20 years; in younger patients the dementia will generally progress at a faster rate, while patients with frontotemporal dementia and motor neurone disease will have a life expectancy of only a few months. Several epidemiological studies report survival data for their cohorts.[6,11] These data suggest that approaching 50% of patients with early onset AD will have died within five years, with a lower survival rate for vascular dementia. There is some evidence to show that the presence of tremor, rigidity or myoclonus is associated with significantly reduced survival at five years after diagnosis.

All of this information is far too much to share in one or even two sessions and needs to be dealt with gradually, in the context of a trusting, supportive relationship, over a period of weeks or months. It is important to give patients the opportunity to discuss their feelings and queries at a later date. They should know that support and help will be ongoing, and that help will be on hand to address both psychological and practical difficulties in the time ahead. The knowledge that there is someone on hand to help with everyday problems, who understands both the person with early onset dementia and carer experience, is in itself usually an enormous help.

Taking a problem-oriented approach is the most effective means of helping the person with early onset dementia and their carer. Helping the person with dementia and their carer to break the illness down into problems that can have a solution, rather than a progressive, degenerative disease, is a much more positive and helpful approach, which, if started early enough in the illness, can significantly relieve stress. It is then possible to see often very distressing symptoms as part of an illness process, which can in turn be addressed in a structured manner. It is also possible to tackle problems not due to dementia, many of which can be remedied.

The other therapeutic aspect of the counselling relationship is in helping the person with dementia and their family come to terms with the changes in their lives, with the losses that have occurred and those still to come. The changes forced upon carers are often considerable, for example changes in financial circumstances with many carers still having large financial commitments such as mortgages, and many carers having to reduce working hours or stop work altogether. In one investigation 90% had financial problems.[9] The same study reported a severe impact on children, with 92% significantly affected by the dementia. Emotional problems, problems at school and conflict with the person with dementia were described. Two major predictors of both increased psychological distress and burden frequently reported in studies are poor marital quality pre-diagnosis and a female carer.

Developing services

Strategic and financial planning should be informed by research and the experiences of people with dementia and their carers, together with clinical experience combined with the evaluation of services.

The Leeds Service has been developing incrementally since 1995 and currently comprises:

- the early onset dementia (EOD) team – with two sessions of time from a consultant psychiatrist, two sessions of time from a consultant clinical psychologist, one full-time community mental health nurse, two half-time social workers, one full-time occupational therapist and a full-time secretary. In addition to community work there is a weekly outpatient clinic.

- Armley Grange Day Centre – run by the Alzheimer's Society, open five days per week, providing 15 places per day specifically for younger people with dementia. Day care has been rated the most valuable service consistently by carers in many surveys in the UK, e.g. Williams et al.[12]

- a group for younger people with dementia and two groups for carers.

- a new outreach service staffed by the Alzheimer's Society, taking referrals from the EOD team to provide additional domiciliary care and help maintain people in their home setting.

- two dedicated beds on a dementia acute ward and agreed access to respite and continuing care beds in a NHS community unit for older people with dementia.

Where specialist provision does not exist then generic services such as home care and Crossroads (a charity providing home-based respite care) are used, as are health services, social services and independent sector services designed for other client groups, e.g. residential and nursing homes for older people with dementia.

Development requires multi-agency working with professionals collaborating across agencies, e.g. clinicians with commissioners and the voluntary sector. Based upon personal experience, I suggest the following ten key messages:[13]

1 Examine current provision.
2 Adapt and develop around existing services.
3 Learn from other people.
4 Plan and be prepared for a long and frustrating process.
5 Set clear aims and objectives.
6 Create political alliances and involve people capable of effecting organisational change.
7 Identify named professionals and 'product champions'.
8 Involve carers – their voice can be very powerful.
9 Involve people with dementia – as above.
10 Action – make a start somewhere! Changing the whole system has to be done in steps.

I have found that even experienced CPNs and specialist registrars find working with younger people extremely challenging, due to the emotional impact of speaking to people of a similar age to themselves about having a diagnosis, together with the complexity of need and severity of behavioural problems. The need for building in supervision and support to staff as well as providing training cannot be overstated. Suggested topics for training include:

- understanding the symptoms and signs of the rarer dementias

- breaking of bad news

- responding to difficult questions.

A comprehensive service model

Any service model should have as its ethos 'joint working' across the whole system of care. A close working relationship between the different service providers is an essential foundation, as is multidisciplinary teamwork, if complex needs are to be met in a coherent and co-ordinated manner. The following issues are critical:

- early and accurate diagnosis

- access for all younger people with dementia to a full range of quality services

- services which reflect the specific needs and circumstances of younger people

- services that are financially justifiable and sustainable.

A study by the Alzheimer's Society found 11 pathways to care[14] and another demonstrated 38 different referral pathways to care.[12] A clear link between neurology services and mental health services goes some way to avoiding the need to negotiate a maze of services.

The Royal College of Psychiatrists proposes that each district should have one named consultant responsible for the service, suggesting old age psychiatrists are best placed to fulfil this role, whilst the task force initiated by the European Federation of Neurological Societies recommends that neurologists should have a clear role in the management of dementia. A recent survey to assess current stated practice in the UK in the diagnosis and management of younger people with dementia confirmed some previously reported differences between old age psychiatrists and neurologists.[15]

It is important to know that neurologists and old age psychiatrists investigate and manage patients differently, especially given that neurologists manage patients without liaison with old age psychiatrists and vice versa. Significantly more old age psychiatrists obtained an independent history from a carer, assessed symptoms of depression and changes in driving performance, arranged community follow-up and prescribed and monitored acetylcholinesterase inhibitor therapy. Significantly more neurologists performed physical examinations and arranged more basic investigations, e.g. plasma viscosity, syphilis serology, EEG as well as more specialist investigations such as lumbar puncture for examination of CSF.

Young patients may be underinvestigated if managed by an old age psychiatrist and may not receive adequate follow-up services if managed solely by a neurologist. The assessment and management of patients with early onset dementia would be greatly improved if the complementary skills of both neurologists and old age psychiatrists were employed in the care of each patient. A joint assessment clinic is probably the best way of facilitating this, but where it does not exist patients should be speedily referred from the diagnostic service to the community mental health team, so as to provide emotional support early. Psychiatrists ought to refer all patients with atypical presentations and those under 50 years old to a neurologist.

The preferred model of care is a named care co-ordinator (from the EOD team) supervising an integrated package of health and social care tailored to individual needs, providing continuity and reviewing changing needs, in other words a Care Programme Approach (CPA) model or equivalent. A community mental health team is the focal point, networked to other services such as day care, respite services and acute hospital services.

There is now a lot of practical experience and an adequate evidence base that demonstrates the need for specialist service provision. This can then streamline the diagnostic process, clarify clinical responsibility, build up expertise, provide continuity and co-ordinate the delivery of care with other agencies.

The future

Two good opportunities that could help younger people with dementia occur at this time: the restructuring of the NHS, involving trusts merging, and the National Service Framework for Older People.[16] The first will produce larger organisations serving larger populations, thus strengthening the case for a specialist service. The NSF for Older People obliges PCTs and local authorities to review, in conjunction with mental health service providers, the current arrangements for the management of dementia in younger people, meaning that this patient group will be included in the NSF for Older People's implementation and joint investment plans developed for each PCT.

Key points

- The practical management of younger people with dementia requires attention to both the clinical challenge, e.g. of diagnosis and psychiatric management, as well as the organisational challenge of how to design and co-ordinate a range of services.
- It is this author's hope and prediction that more new services will be set up and that the existing knowledge base will fully inform clinical practice and management.

References

1   Alzheimer's Disease Society (1996) *Younger People with Dementia: a review and Strategy.* ADS, London

2   Harvey R (1998) *Young Onset Dementia: epidemiology, clinical symptoms, family burden, support and outcome.* Imperial College School of Medicine, London.

3   Ferran J, Wilson K, Doran M *et al.* (1996) The early-onset dementias: a study of clinical characteristics and service use. *International Journal of Geriatric Psychiatry.* **11**: 863–9.

4   Donaldson C, Tarrier N and Burns A (1997) The impact of the symptoms of dementia on care-givers. *British Journal of Psychiatry.* **170**: 62–8.

5   Teri L (1997) Behaviour and care-giver burden: behavioural problems in patients with Alzheimer disease and its association with care-giver distress. *Alzheimer Disease and Associated Disorders.* **11**: S35–S38.

6   Newens A, Forster D, Kay D *et al.* (1993) Clinically diagnosed presenile dementia of the Alzheimer type in the Northern region: ascertainment, prevalence, incidence and survival. *Psychological Medicine.* **23**: 631–44.

7   Cruts M, Vanduijn CM, Backhovens H *et al.* (1998) Estimation of the genetic contribution of presenilin-1 and -2 mutations in a population-based study of pre-senile Alzheimer's disease. *Human Molecular Genetics.* **7**: 43–51.

8   Hodges JR (ed.) (2001) *Early Onset Dementia: a multidisciplinary approach.* Oxford University Press, Oxford.

9   Luscombe G, Brodaty H and Freeth S (1998) Younger people with dementia: diagnostic issues, effects on carers and use of services. *International Journal of Geriatric Psychiatry.* **13**: 323–30.

10 Nott P and Fleminger J (1975) Presenile dementia: the difficulties of early diagnosis. *Acta Psychiatrica Scandinavica.* **51**: 210–17.

11   Whalley L, Thomas B, McGonigal G *et al.* (1995) Epidemiology of pre-senile Alzheimer's disease in Scotland (1974–1988). *British Journal of Psychiatry.* **167**: 728–31.

12   Williams T, Dearden AM and Cameron IC (2001) From pillar to post: a study of younger people with dementia. *Psychiatric Bulletin.* **25**: 384–7.

13   Alzheimer's Disease Society (2001) *Younger People with Dementia: a guide to service development and provision.* ADS, London.

14   Fuhrmann R (1997) *Early Onset Dementia in the Brighton, Hove and Lewes Area: prevalence and service needs.* Alzheimer's Disease Society, Brighton.

15   Cordery R, Harvey R, Frost C *et al.* (2002) National survey to assess current practices in the diagnosis and management of young people with dementia. *International Journal of Geriatric Psychiatry.* **17**: 124–7.

16   Department of Health (2001) *National Service Framework for Older People.* DoH, London.

Further reading

Cox S and Keady J (eds) (1999) *Younger People with Dementia: planning, practice and development.* Jessica Kingsley, London.

Neary D (1994) Classification of the dementias. *Reviews in Clinical Gerontology.* **4**: 131–40.

Royal College of Psychiatrists (2000) *Services for Younger People with Alzheimer's Disease and Other Dementias.* Council Report No. 77. Royal College of Psychiatrists, London.

Williams R, Barrett K and Muth Z (eds) (1997) *Mental Health Services: heading for better care – commissioning and providing mental health services for people with Huntington's disease, acquired brain injury and early-onset dementia.* NHS Health Advisory Service thematic review. HMSO, London.

Williams T, Cameron I, Dearden T *et al.* (1999) *From Pillar to Post: early-onset dementia in Leeds – prevalence, experience and service need.* Leeds Health Authority.

14

Legal aspects of management

Shabir Musa

People with dementia present with various clinical features. These include decline in cognition, intellectual functioning, reasoning ability, judgement and insight. Legal issues, mainly related to capacity, arise from these features.

Capacity

Capacity is a legal concept. Medical practitioners are frequently asked to give opinions about an individual's capacity. Psychiatrists are usually consulted about capacity issues in complex cases and when someone is suspected of suffering, or is suffering, from a mental disorder like dementia. In disputed cases of capacity, the courts make the final decision.

In English law, an adult has the right to make decisions affecting their own life, whether the reasons for the choice are rational, irrational, unknown or even non-existent. This right remains even if the outcome of the decision might be detrimental to the individual. However, such a right to self-determination is meaningful only if the individual is appropriately informed, has the ability (capacity) to make the decision and is free to decide without coercion.[1] An adult is presumed to have the capacity until the contrary is proven, and a person who legally lacks capacity remains in that state until the contrary is proven.

Definition of capacity

There is at present no statutory definition of capacity. In 1995, the Law Commission for England and Wales completed a major review of the law in relation to mental incapacity[2] and presented a draft bill to the Lord Chancellor. The Law Commission's definition of incapacity is summarised in Box 14.1.

Box 14.1   The Law Commission's definition of incapacity[2]

A person is without capacity if at the material time they are:
- unable by reason of mental disability to make a decision on the matter in question. The person is unable to:
  - understand relevant information

> - retain this information
> - make a decision based on information given
> - unable to communicate a choice on that matter because he or she is unconscious or for any other reason.

The Law Commission also makes the following points. Firstly, adults who do not have a mental disorder cannot be considered to be without capacity. Secondly, 'mental disability' is defined as 'any disability or disorder of the mind or brain, whether permanent or temporary, which results in a disturbance or impairment of mental functioning'. Thirdly, decision making capacity might vary depending on the subject of the decision and it might change over time. It depends not only on the decision maker but also on the characteristics of the decision, including the complexity and the way it is presented. Fourthly, assessment of capacity should be based on the 'balance of probabilities'.

There are various legal tests of capacity which need to be applied depending on the specific capacity that is being assessed. To find out more about these various legal tests of capacity, the reader is referred to the publication by the British Medical Association.[3]

Capacity to deal with financial affairs

Powers of attorney

A power of attorney is a deed by which one person (the *donor*) gives another person (the *attorney*) the authority to act in the donor's name and on their behalf in relation to the donor's property and financial affairs. It is possible to choose more than one attorney. If more than one attorney is chosen then they could act either jointly (that is, they must all act together and cannot act separately) or jointly and severally (that is, they can all act together but they can also act separately if they wish). A power of attorney can be specific or general. If it is specific, the attorney only has the authority to do the things specified by the donor in the power. If it is general, the attorney has the authority to do anything that the donor can lawfully do with their property and affairs. i.e. the attorney is able to deal with money or property and may be able to sell the donor's house.

There are two types of powers of attorney.

Ordinary power of attorney

The test of capacity, which a person must satisfy in order to make an ordinary power of attorney, is that the donor understands the nature and effect of what they are doing. An ordinary power of attorney tends to be used as a temporary expedient; for example where the donor is going abroad for several months and needs someone to look after various legal or financial transactions during their absence. Although the legal form completed by the donor is usually simple, it is generally advisable to seek legal advice. An ordinary power of attorney ceases to have effect if the donor becomes mentally incapable, for example if they develop significant dementia. The donor or the attorney can cancel an ordinary power of attorney at any time.

Enduring power of attorney (EPA)

Enduring powers became available in England and Wales in March 1986, when the Enduring Powers of Attorney Act 1985 came into force. This Act provides a procedure whereby power of attorney continues to operate after the donor has become mentally incapable.

Procedure: the donor and the proposed attorney sign an enduring power of attorney form in the presence of an independent witness. A second witness is only necessary if the form is not signed by the donor personally, but by someone else in the donor's presence and at their direction. The donor should be capable of understanding the information in Box 14.2 in order to create an enduring power of attorney.

Box 14.2   Capacity to make an enduring power of attorney

The person creating an enduring power of attorney should understand the following information:

- If such be the terms of the power, the attorney will be able to assume complete authority over the donor's affairs.
- If such be the terms of the power, the attorney will be able to do anything with the donor's property which the donor could have done.
- The authority will continue if the donor should be or should become mentally incapable.
- If the donor becomes mentally incapable, the power will be irrevocable without confirmation by the Court of Protection.

Solicitors are advised that when a donor is of borderline capacity, that the power is witnessed or approved by a medical practitioner who should record their findings. Unless the enduring power specifically states that it will not come into force until the donor is mentally incapacitated, the power is 'live'. The enduring power can be used concurrently with the donor. When the donor becomes mentally incapable of managing and administering their affairs, then the attorney should apply to register the enduring power with the Court of Protection. The donor and nearest relatives have the right to object to the registration of the power. Once the power has been registered, it cannot be cancelled or revoked by the donor. The Court of Protection can remove an unsatisfactory attorney.

In its report, the Law Commission (1995) recommended the creation of a new power of attorney called a 'continuing power of attorney'. This would make it possible to appoint an attorney to take decisions about the donor's personal welfare and medical treatment, as well as the person's property and financial affairs. However, this would require new legislation.

Court of Protection

Where a person who has not made an enduring power of attorney becomes incapable, by reason of mental disorder, of managing and administering their property and affairs, then it may be necessary to apply to the Court of Protection for the appointment of a *receiver* to deal with the day-to-day management of the person's affairs.

History

The origins of the Court of Protection go back to the Middle Ages when the Crown assumed the responsibility of managing the affairs of the mentally ill and mentally handicapped. It is an office of the Supreme Court and its head is called the Master. People whose affairs are managed by the Court are known as 'patients'. The Court's powers and procedures are governed by Part VII of the Mental Health Act 1983 and by the Court of Protection Rules 1984. Its administrative functions are now carried out by the Public Trust Office. The Public Trust Office has a Protection Division, which deals with external receivers, and a Management Division, which acts as a receiver when no one else can be found.

Procedure

An application is made to the Court, usually by a close relative, solicitor or an officer of the local authority. This must be accompanied by details of the individual's family circumstances and financial affairs. The Court also requires medical evidence. This is provided by a registered medical practitioner who completes a medical certificate known as Form CP3, confirming that the patient is incapable, by reason of mental disorder, of managing and administering their property and affairs. The Court, in consultation with the Royal College of Psychiatrists and the British Medical Association, has prepared guidance notes to assist medical practitioners in completing the form. Relatives or the patient, at a formal hearing, where a receiver is usually appointed, can raise objections to the process.

Relatives are usually appointed as receiver, but in complex cases, or where there may be a conflict of interest, professional people may be more appropriate. The receiver is accountable to the Court for any decisions that are taken, and is expected to visit the patient and be consulted about significant changes in their care. The Court monitors the performance of receivers. There is power to displace an unsuitable receiver. The Court can revoke the authority if convinced by medical evidence that Court of Protection is no longer required as the patient has regained capacity to manage their own affairs. If the Court requires a specialist opinion about a person's mental capacity, it may instruct one of the Lord Chancellor's Medical Visitors to provide a report.

The Law Commission in 1995 recommended in its report that the powers of the Court of Protection are extended to include making decisions about the patient's personal welfare and medical treatment.

Appointeeship

The appointeeship system enables another individual, known as an *appointee*, to receive and administer social security benefits and allowances on behalf of a mentally incapable person. Appointeeship is governed by Regulation 33 of the Social Security (Claims and Payments) Regulations 1987. Medical evidence of the claimant's inability to manage their own affairs may be requested.

The Secretary of State can revoke an appointment at any time, and there is no right of appeal to a tribunal against the Secretary of State's refusal to appoint a particular individual as appointee or against the revocation of such an appointment. Appointees have no authority to deal with the claimant's capital. Appointeeship automatically lapses as soon as receivership is made by the Court of Protection. Enduring power of attorney does not affect appointeeship, although the attorney will become the appointee if necessary.

Capacity to make a will

A will is a document in which the maker (*testator* or *testatrix*) appoints an executor to deal with their affairs when the person dies. The degree of understanding, which the law requires a person making a will to have, is known as *testamentary capacity*. Testamentary capacity should be present both when giving instructions for the preparation of the will and at the time of execution or signing of the will. A greater degree of mental capacity is likely to be required when making a complex will in comparison to a simple will.

The criteria listed in Box 14.3 should be assessed in deciding whether an individual has testamentary capacity.

Box 14.3   Testamentary capacity

An individual making a will should:
- understand the nature of the act and its effects
- understand the nature and extent of the property being disposed
- be able to distinguish and compare potential beneficiaries
- be free from an abnormal state of mind.

A person with mental disorder may legitimately make a will, provided the mental disorder does not influence any of the criteria relevant to the making of the will. Old age psychiatrists and GPs are most likely to be asked to give their opinions as to testamentary capacity in cases of presumed or established dementia. Solicitors are advised that when drawing up a will for an elderly person or someone who is seriously ill, to ensure that the will is witnessed or approved by a medical practitioner. The medical practitioner should record their examination and findings.

The capacity to revoke a will is the same as the capacity of making a will in the first place. A will is automatically revoked when the person gets married.

Statutory wills

If a person is both (a) incapable, by reason of mental disorder, of managing and administering their property and affairs, and (b) incapable of making a valid will, an application can be made to the Court of Protection for a statutory will to be drawn up and executed on the person's behalf. The Court requires medical evidence of both types of incapacity. The Court is obliged to make a will, consistent with the one the patient would have made for themselves, within reason, and with competent legal advice.

Dementia and driving

It is the duty of the driving licence holder or the applicant to notify the Driver and Vehicle Licensing Authority of any medical condition which may affect safe driving. DVLA must be notified as soon as a diagnosis of dementia is made. In early dementia when sufficient skills are retained and progression is slow, a licence may be issued subject to annual review. A formal driving assessment may be necessary. It is extremely difficult to assess driving ability in those with dementia.

There are some circumstances in which the licence holder cannot, or will not, inform the DVLA of a significant medical condition which may affect safe driving. Under these circumstances the General Medical Council has issued clear guidelines. These are:

- The DVLA is legally responsible for deciding if a person is medically unfit to drive. They need to know when driving licence holders have a condition that may, now or in the future, affect their safety as a driver.

- Therefore, where patients have such conditions, the doctor should make sure that the patients understand that the condition may impair their ability to drive. If a patient is incapable of understanding this advice, for example because of dementia, the doctor should inform the DVLA immediately. The doctor should explain to patients that they have a legal duty to inform the DVLA about the condition.

- If patients refuse to accept the diagnosis or effect of the condition on their ability to drive, the doctor can suggest that the patients seek a second opinion. The patients should be advised not to drive until the second opinion has been obtained.

- If patients continue to drive when they are not fit to do so, every reasonable effort should be made to persuade them to stop. This may include telling their next of kin.

- If the patient continues to drive contrary to medical advice, the doctor should disclose relevant medical information immediately, in confidence, to the medical advisor at the DVLA.

- Before giving information to the DVLA, the doctor should inform the patient of their decision to do so. Once the DVLA has been informed, the doctor should also write to the patient to confirm that a disclosure has been made.[4]

When the DVLA is notified about any relevant medical condition, the medical advisor can take several possible courses of action. They may request more information about the patient's current state of health from the GP or hospital doctor. The patient may be requested to undergo a medical examination by a doctor appointed by the DVLA. In some circumstances, the medical advisor may require the patient to be examined by a clinical psychologist. If a decision to revoke the driving licence is taken, this is communicated to the patient by letter. The individual has the legal right to appeal against the decision, but such appeals are rarely successful.

Capacity to consent to medical treatment

An adult is presumed to have capacity until the contrary is proven. Most people with early dementia are capable of giving valid consent to common medical treatments. It is the personal responsibility of any doctor proposing to treat a patient to judge whether the patient has the capacity to give a valid consent. The capacity required to make a decision about medical treatment was discussed in the case of *Re C (Adult: Refusal of Treatment)*.[5] The High Court held that an adult has capacity to consent (or refuse consent) to medical treatment if the criteria listed in Box 14.4 are met.

Box 14.4   Capacity to consent to medical treatment

An individual has capacity if they can:
- understand and retain the relevant information
- believe the information
- weigh that information in the balance to arrive at a choice.

To demonstrate capacity, individuals should be able to:

- understand in simple language what the medical treatment is, its purpose and nature and why it is being proposed

- understand the principal benefits, risks and alternatives

- understand what the consequences will be of not receiving the proposed treatment

- retain the information for long enough to make an effective decision, and
- make a free choice.

Advance statements

If an individual is found to lack capacity, then reference should be made to any advance statement the person may have made. Advance statements are also sometimes referred to as 'advance directives' or 'advance refusals' or 'living wills'. Advance statements are declarations whereby competent people make known their views on what should happen if they lose the capacity to make decisions for themselves. This allows people to state which treatments they would or would not want if they become seriously ill and no longer have the mental capacity to make decisions. Advance statements can take a variety of forms, ranging from general lists of life values and preferences to specific requests or refusals. They can be written or oral.

Advance statements about healthcare decisions are currently valid under common law. Where a patient has lost capacity to make a decision but has a valid advance statement refusing life-prolonging treatment, this must be respected. A valid advance refusal of treatment has the same legal authority as a contemporaneous refusal, and legal action could be taken against a doctor who provides treatment in the face of a valid refusal.

The test for capacity to make an advance statement about medical treatment is similar to that for capacity to make a contemporaneous medical decision. In order for an advance statement to be valid, the patient must have been competent when the statement was made, must be acting free from pressure and must have been offered sufficient, accurate information to make an informed decision. It is recommended that advance statements be updated regularly, usually every three years, to indicate that they truly reflect the person's current views.

Benefits

Firstly, the patient benefits as they can be sure that their wishes will be respected. Secondly, doctors benefit as they will no longer have to guess what the patient would have wanted, and are free of conflicting views from relatives. Thirdly, relatives and friends benefit as they have documentary evidence of the patient's wishes and are freed from the responsibility of making decisions on someone else's behalf.

Best interests

Individuals who lack capacity to give consent to medical treatment and have not made an advance statement should be treated under the principle of 'best interests'. As a matter of good practice it is advisable to obtain a second opinion from another doctor in cases where a complex decision is contemplated.

When treating individuals in their best interests, consideration should be given to the:

- past and present wishes of the individual

- need to maximise the person's participation in the decision

- views of others as to the person's wishes and feelings

- need to adopt the course of action that is least restrictive to the individual's freedom.

Mental Health Act (1983)

The Bournewood case

Most people with dementia, including those who lack capacity, are treated in hospital informally. People with dementia who lack capacity and do not show any dissent to be hospitalised or to receive treatment are admitted informally under the common law doctrine of necessity. This point was further clarified in the recent Bournewood case.[6] This case involved HL, a 48-year-old man with autism who had spent many years in Bournewood Hospital, Surrey. In 1994, he went to live with Mr and Mrs E, who cared for him and treated him as one of their family. In July 1997, while attending a day centre he became agitated and was readmitted *informally* to Bournewood Hospital. His admission was challenged in court in October 1997 which ruled that he was illegally detained and that he could be legally detained only if he were admitted formally under the Mental Health Act 1983. The Court of Appeal upheld this decision on 2 December 1997. These rulings meant that all patients in hospital who lacked capacity to consent to treatment, even if they did not dissent either to remain in hospital or to receive treatment, had to be detained under the Mental Health Act 1983. The judgement of the Court of Appeal was later overturned in the House of Lords on 25 June 1998 and the situation effectively returned to what it was before.

Since the Bournewood case, there has been a lot of debate about the legal and ethical issues regarding the treatment of people who lack capacity to consent to treatment. It is generally felt that there is a gap in the current Mental Health Act as regards treatment of vulnerable, incapacitated patients. People with dementia who lack capacity and are treated informally are not afforded the same safeguards and legal rights as compared to those incapacitated patients who are treated under the Mental Health Act 1983. It is proposed in the White Paper on Reforming the Mental Health Act[7] that patients with long-term incapacity in hospitals and residential/nursing homes (but not those at home or in other settings), while not being subject to a compulsory order, will be subject to a statutory process whereby treatment plans must be written and the approval of a second-opinion doctor sought.

Patients with dementia may become subject to various sections of the Mental Health Act 1983. A brief account will be given of the more commonly applied sections of the Act relevant to people with dementia. For a detailed account of all the possible sections of the Act that are applicable to patients with dementia, the reader is referred to the *Mental Health Act Manual*.[8]

Section 5 (2): doctor's holding power

An informal inpatient who wishes to leave hospital may be detained for up to 72 hours if the doctor believes an application should be made for compulsory admission under the Act. This requires a single medical recommendation by the doctor in charge of the patient's care, or their nominated deputy. It is usual to consider a change to a Section 2 or 3 order as soon as possible.

Section 2: assessment order

Criteria

Section 2 provides that a person may be detained under the Act for a period of up to 28 days on the grounds that the person:

- is suffering from a mental disorder of a nature or degree which warrants detention in hospital for assessment or assessment followed by treatment
- ought to be detained in the interests of the patient's own health or safety or with a view to the protection of others.

Procedure

This requires:

- *application* by the patient's nearest relative, or an approved social worker who must have seen the patient within the last 14 days. The approved social worker should, so far as it is practicable, consult the nearest relative
- *medical recommendations* by two doctors, one of whom must be approved under Section 12 of the Act. If the medical recommendations are performed separately, then they should be done within five days of each other.

Section 3: treatment order

Criteria

Section 3 provides that a person may be detained under the Act for an initial period of up to 6 months on the grounds that:

- the person is suffering from mental illness, severe mental impairment, psycho-pathic disorder or mental impairment and the mental disorder is of a nature or degree which makes it appropriate for them to receive medical treatment in hospital

- in the case of psychopathic disorder or mental impairment, such treatment is likely to alleviate or prevent a deterioration in the person's condition

- it is necessary for the health or safety of the person or for the protection of others that the person should receive such treatment and it cannot be provided unless they are detained under Section 3.

Procedure

This requires:

- *application* by the patient's nearest relative or an approved social worker. The social worker must, if practicable, consult the nearest relative before making an application and cannot proceed if the nearest relative objects

- *medical recommendations* similar to those for Section 2. In addition, the recommendations must state the particular grounds for the doctor's opinion, specifying whether any other methods of dealing with the patient are available and, if so, why they are not appropriate. The doctor must specify one of the four forms of mental disorder.

The order may be renewed on the first occasion for a further six months and subsequently for a year at a time.

Section 7: Guardianship order

The purpose of guardianship is to enable patients to receive community care where it cannot be provided without the use of compulsory powers. It provides an authoritative framework for working with a patient, with a minimum constraint, to achieve as independent a life as possible within the community.

Procedure

The application, medical recommendations, duration and renewal are similar to those for Section 3. The guardian is usually the local social services department. Sometimes a private individual is appointed as the guardian. The guardian has a number of powers and these are detailed in Box 14.5.

Box 14.5 Powers of guardianship

The guardian has the power to require:
- the patient to reside at a place specified by the guardian
- the patient to attend places specified by the guardian for the purpose of medical treatment, occupation, education or training
- access to be given to the patient's residence to any doctor, approved social worker or other person so specified by the guardian.

Limitations

Guardianship does not give a specific power of conveyance. Therefore, if the patient refused to attend a clinic or day hospital for treatment, or refused to go and reside at a place specified by the guardian, then it would not be possible to force the patient to attend or go. There is also no power to force entry into the patient's home, if the patient refuses access. For guardianship to be successful, a degree of co-operation is required from the patient.

Conclusions

Various medico-legal issues arise in people suffering from dementia as it is a chronic degenerative illness. There is a progressive decline in cognition, intellectual functioning, reasoning ability, judgement and insight in these patients. Issues in relation to capacity occur most frequently. In such situations, there are various legal tests of capacity which need to be applied depending on the specific capacity that is being assessed.

Key points

- Capacity is a legal concept.
- An adult is presumed to have capacity until the contrary is proven.
- Most people with early dementia are capable of giving valid consent to common medical treatments.
- People with dementia who lack capacity and do not show any dissent to being hospitalised or to receive treatment should be admitted informally.
- Advance statements about healthcare decisions are currently valid under common law.
- A person with mental disorder may legitimately make a will, provided the mental disorder does not influence any of the criteria relevant to making of the will.
- The DVLA is legally responsible for deciding a person's medical fitness to drive.

References

1 Grisso T (1986) *Evaluating Competencies: forensic assessments and instruments.* Plenum, New York.
2 Law Commission (1995) *Mental Incapacity: a summary of the Law Commission's recommendations* (LC 231). HMSO, London.
3 British Medical Association and Law Society (1990) *Assessment of Mental Incapacity: guidance for doctors and lawyers.* BMA, London.
4 Driver and Vehicle Licensing Authority (2002) *At-a-Glance Guide to the Current Medical Standards of Fitness to Drive for Medical Practitioners.* DVLA, Swansea.
5 *Re C (Adult: Refusal of Treatment)* (1994) 1WLR 290.
6 *R v Bournewood Community and Mental Health NHS Trust, ex parte L* (1998) 3 A11ER 289.
7 Department of Health (2000) *Reforming the Mental Health Act.* HMSO, London.
8 Jones R (2001) *Mental Health Act Manual.* Sweet and Maxwell, London.

15
Spiritual aspects of dementia

Daphne Wallace

Spirituality

Spirituality is a concept that has varied interpretations. In order to talk about spiritual aspects of dementia, I feel that it is important to start with the working definition that I shall use throughout (see Box 15.1). John Swinton[1] devotes the whole of his first chapter to this issue in a book exploring the spiritual aspects of mental healthcare. It is a common assumption that 'spiritual' and 'religious' are interchangeable. In care plans and assessment of needs it seems often to be seen as an optional extra. Krishna Mohan, in Consciousness and its Transformation,[2] comments: 'Though spirituality traditionally has been considered to be exclusively the domain of religion, it is now being conceptualised in terms that have no particular relationship to theology, and is at the same time being accepted as practically and intellectually respectable'.

Box 15.1   Definition of spirituality

Spirituality may usefully be defined thus:

Spirituality is regarded as a basic characteristic of all people, which is vital to health and well-being. It is a universal search for meaning and purpose, which is an essential part of being human.

   For those with a religious faith, their relationship with God may be one of those relationships that give meaning and purpose to their lives.

Spiritual care

In the past, spiritual care, however understood, was considered the responsibility of the hospital chaplain, minister of religion, priest or religious leader – it was left to the 'expert'.[3]

   With the change to the concept of whole-person care there is increasing awareness that spiritual well-being is relevant and important. Attention to spiritual needs leads to a better quality of life. Meeting them is not an add-on 'icing on the cake' but an integral part of whole-person care. Recognition of the person-hood of the individual is vital.

As pointed out by Kitwood,[4] for the greater part of the period in which dementia has existed as a clinical category, the subjectivity of those affected has been almost totally disregarded. Despite the writing of Alison Froggatt[5] when she drew attention to this area, this was not really followed up, and if so, only with those with milder cognitive disability.

For some time concern has been expressed for those with dementia. The tendency to see people with advanced dementia as non-persons is still pervasive and, despite much work to change the situation, as a group their spiritual needs tend to be particularly neglected. Reverend Eileen Shamy, a Methodist minister from New Zealand, started a ministry for those with dementia. This was partly informed by her experience of looking after her mother with dementia for 12 years. Writing with Alison Froggatt[6] and in her own book *More than Body, Brain and Breath,*[7] she describes this experience.

Describing the last days of her mother's 12-year journey through Alzheimer's disease, she says:

> Some days she forgot who I was and some days she confused me with her younger sister ... At the end, only three days before her death, out of the dull grey of memory loss and confusion she said to me, firmly and clear-eyed, 'God never forgets us. Remember that, dear!' At that moment her suffering and my weary questioning was shot through with light. The whole devastating experience began to acquire new meaning. I knew then that nothing had been lost and that in the end all would be harvest. I am now committed, and others with me, to an unmapped journey, sustained by grace and deep gut prayer. It is a journey towards holistic care for people with Alzheimer's disease and related dementias, in which the spiritual dimension of care is given as much respectful attention as the physical, emotional and social dimensions.

Person-centred care

Tom Kitwood's seminal work on person-centred care for those with dementia has also altered many misperceptions of the needs of people with dementia. There are many publications from the Bradford Dementia Group of Bradford University, well represented by him in *The New Culture of Dementia Care*[8] and *Dementia Reconsidered.*[4] As he pointed out, there is an 'old' and a 'new' culture of dementia care. The 'old' is well illustrated by an account of an agency's approach to a day centre, wishing to promote awareness about Alzheimer's disease. They asked for some photographs of clients for publicity purposes. Permission was sought and granted and the photographs duly taken and sent. They were rejected because they did not show the disturbed and agonised characteristics that people with dementia 'ought' to show. Stirling University Dementia Services Development Centre has also published material about the needs of the elderly with dementia, including spiritual needs (see below).

Communication

Malcolm Goldsmith, during his time at Stirling, did research into communication with those with dementia, published as *Hearing the Voice of People with Dementia*.[9]

John Killick has developed his skills as writer and poet to help those with dementia communicate, and has produced books of 'assisted' writings[10,11] where he writes down the things said to him in conversation when visiting as writer in residence to Westminster Health Care and the Stirling Dementia Services Development Centre. As Sue Benson, Editor of *Journal of Dementia Care*, says in the foreword to the collection published as *You are Words*:[10]

> John Killick's work has made two very special contributions to the cause of good practice in dementia care. Giving time and concentrated attention to an individual, listening carefully to what they say, tells each person with dementia they are valued, that they are of interest and worth. The further step of writing down what is said powerfully underlines that statement of worth.

His work has shown that even those who are severely affected by dementia, who care staff believe to be incapable of communicating, can, with attention and confidence in the listener, communicate with great clarity and insight.

The current situation

Unfortunately, despite all this valuable work, many people with dementia languish in institutions with little attention paid to their individual needs, wishes and personalities. It is vital that as well as attempts to ensure sufficient space, good food, privacy and healthcare, the needs of the individual person are not ignored. Such small things can make a vital difference to the well-being of the individual. Eileen Shamy[7] gives a telling example of simple needs not met (see Case Study 15.1).

Case Study 15.1

Eileen Shamy describes a sequence of events with her mother:

As an example of the deprivation this can cause, I think of my mother who had always been a talented needlewoman and craftsperson. Her hands were never idle. When she went into a nursing home because she needed 24-hour care she was still crocheting. She crocheted squares for Afghan quilts and her work, even then, was some of the most perfectly executed I have ever seen. She took pleasure in the colours, arranging them harmoniously and crocheting the squares together. That she found the work satisfying was obvious. It seemed to me that the fact that her hands were always busy was the reason she seldom wandered or showed any impatience with being confined to the house and garden.

One weekend when it happened that I could not visit, she dropped her hook and could not find it. All that day, on and off – I was told afterwards – she picked up her work and asked for her crochet hook. No one thought it important to look for it and the weekend staff did not know that she had a spare hook in her room. She still had her work-basket in the lounge on Monday when I visited again. Immediately I noticed her still hands. I picked up the partly completed quilt and she began to cry. Why was she crying? A passing regular staff remarked, 'She hasn't crocheted all day. Weekend staff told us that she was very agitated most of Saturday and Sunday. The cook said that she had lost her crochet hook.'

I went to fetch the spare hook from her room and placed it in her hands. She looked bewildered so I took it and crocheted a few stitches. I told her that she was much, much better at this than I was. But when I placed the hook in her hand she held it awkwardly and poked it aimlessly, not even connecting it to the wool. Silently she put it down and folded her hands. She never picked it up again. It was a kind of dying. I grieved for her loss.

Why had no one thought to fetch her spare hook? If I had been well enough to visit her that weekend, would she still have been crocheting? If she had dropped her soup spoon, someone most certainly would have replaced that for her.

I was right to grieve. She remained sad and restless and her little hands stiffened without the exercise. Worse, another resource for nourishing her spiritual well-being was lost to her.

The recently published *National Minimum Standards for Care Homes for Older People*,[12] which form the basis on which the National Care Standards Commission will inspect and regulate homes, only mentions spiritual needs in the context of dying and death (Standard 11). Unfortunately, the Alzheimer's Society's recently published *Quality Dementia Care in Care Homes: person-centred standards*[13] does little to remedy this omission and the suggested further reading does not include any of the many recent publications relating to spiritual care of those with dementia. Much disappointment has been expressed with regard to the standards, not least by the Coalition for Quality in Care, which has brought together over 50 individuals and groups who have expressed their disappointment. The guidance focuses on physical standards rather than the needs and interests of those cared for. A recent article in the *Church Times* by Barry Hope (p. 21, 19 April 2002) draws attention to this and stresses the need for 'an attitude of treating others as you would wish to be treated yourself', but again does not mention spiritual needs or person-centred care and the work that has been done in these areas during the last ten years. Much work has been done by Tom Kitwood and the Bradford University Dementia Group, Stirling University Dementia Services Development Centre and a number of Christian organisations, including CCOA Dementia Working Group, Methodist Homes, Trinity Care and Faith in Elderly People, Leeds. As Alison Johnson[14] pointed out, there is a need for sensitive care with recognition that people with dementia retain their personhood and that those with failing mental powers need in every way to be treated as persons, just as we would like to be treated.

The spiritual needs of those with dementia are not only important in institutional care. Many old people live in the community, and half of those over 75 live alone.[15] Relatives may also fail to understand their dear ones' spiritual needs. Person-centred care can just as easily be applied at home and usually is, but, importantly, good care in a residential home should not be hampered by relatives (see Case Studies 15.2 and 15.3).

Case Study 15.2

A retired nurse lived in a residential home. Putting on her make-up first thing in the day had always been an important part of her routine.

One day her daughter visited and her make-up was less perfectly put on than usual. With a comment that her mother was no longer capable of doing it properly, she took away all her mother's make-up items. For two or three days the resident searched for her make-up, becoming increasingly upset and agitated. Eventually the staff bought her some replacement items and she was pleased to resume her daily routine.

The daughter presumably could not cope with the lessening of competence in her mother.

Case Study 15.3

An elderly patient in a hospital continuing-care ward had a number of family photographs near his bed. One day the relatives removed them all. Eventually, on enquiry, the staff discovered that they had been worried about the danger of the glass in the frames.

Unfortunately, they therefore removed his special personal effects and his one contact with his family when they were not actually visiting.

Spiritual care: medical

Psychiatrists have had problems with spiritual aspects of care. David Crossley, in an editorial in the *British Journal of Psychiatry*,[16] says: 'It comes as a surprise that psychiatrists should be so reticent in their inquiry into this aspect of their patients' emotional and cognitive experiences.' Since his editorial and the earlier comments by Andrew Sims,[17] the Spirituality Interest Group in the Royal College of Psychiatrists has been founded and grown significantly in membership. As I have outlined, religious belief is only one expression of the spirituality of the person.

Scott Peck[18] alludes to the criticism of atheist friends that 'religion is a crutch for old people as they face the mystery, the terror of their death'. Later in the same book he talks about 'Our unique human capacity for change and transformation is reflected in our human spirituality'. In an epilogue to the book he remarks:

> Although perhaps recently underestimated, the psychodynamic and social aspects of mental illness have held a respected place in the history of American psychiatry. Its spiritual aspects, however, have not. Psychiatry has not only neglected but actively ignored the issue of spirituality.

He then alludes to the confusion between 'spirituality' and 'religion' and consequent misinterpretation which has contributed to this neglect.

Spiritual care: nursing

Over the last few years much work has been done in hospitals on care planning. This has more recently been introduced as standard practice in residential and nursing homes. Recent work has been directed towards developing care plans which will ensure that good quality care is delivered in such settings. Good quality care takes into account the physical, emotional and spiritual dimensions of health. Most care-givers are familiar with recognising, implementing and evaluating physical and emotional care; the spiritual aspect is more difficult to identify and assess. Mary Nathan, speaking at a meeting of the Spirituality Interest Group of the Royal College of Psychiatrists, described work she has done at the West London Mental Health Trust studying the perceptions of spiritual care in patients and the nurses who care for them. She also looked at whether or not mental health nurses feel sufficiently competent to assess and provide spiritual care to their clients. She has also looked at the possible barriers to provision of spiritual care.

Her findings showed that nurses had a lack of clarity with the concept of spirituality, which was most often thought of as related to meeting patients' religious needs. They identified a lack of training in this area and were unclear as to who should be responsible for this aspect of care.

Patients, in contrast, related spiritual care more to qualities of life and recovery. Nurses demonstrated a lack of confidence and expertise regarding spiritual care but did express an interest in undertaking training when provided. Two of the main barriers identified were the lack of clarity of the concept and the confusion of religion and spirituality. Education was seen as an important means of overcoming barriers and using positive attitudes towards self and others in implementing care interventions that address the whole person.

Care in many contexts such as hospital, residential and nursing homes, and at home with home care has become so task-orientated that there seems to be no time left for relatedness. How often in the past has a particular home help or care assistant become a real friend to the person with dementia? Real mourning follows the death or removal of the particular carer. With the time-conscious, task-orientated carer, will this ever be the same? One hopes so or our own lives in later dependency will be bleak indeed.

Care plan guidance

A recent publication has drawn together much work on meeting the spiritual needs of those with dementia into a set of guidelines for care staff.[19] Two project workers, Gaynor Hammond and Laraine Moffitt, from Leeds and Newcastle respectively, have written this to 'help staff understand the nature of spiritual needs and how to meet them, and arises out of work with care of older people, especially people with dementia'. The booklet aims to cultivate an approach which weaves spiritual care throughout the whole of care giving. In this way it exemplifies Tom Kitwood's concept of person-centred care for the whole person in the entirety of their care needs. As they point out in the conclusion of the booklet, 'By acknowledging the spiritual dimension within all care practice, it may be easier for staff to justify why bathing a certain resident took longer today than usual – it may be that today the bathing met a need at the deepest level'.

We accept unquestioningly that bathing a young child may be a time of very important interpersonal communication. Why is it assumed that this possibility disappears as we become adults? Many have written about the deep spiritual understanding and responsiveness in those with severe learning disabilities. Why do we assume that the onset of dementia immediately destroys this essential part of human existence? Much that has been written about person-centred care for those with dementia applies to everyone in a care-receiving situation. Those with dementia are the least able to express their needs and thus have become a focus for attention. It is sad that in the early part of the twenty-first century there are still many being 'cared for' in situations where their spiritual needs are ignored or not even acknowledged.

Religious practice

The Prince of Wales has pointed to the irony of asking a patient on admission to hospital to which religion they belong and then ignoring all that their religion may bring them in terms of how they understand and cope with illness. Religious observance may be one way to meet a spiritual need but there may be others, even for a person of faith. Severe dementia, however, does not prevent a person responding appropriately and with great benefit to religious observance. Rituals and symbols are important but those visiting in this capacity must be prepared to be flexible and expect the unexpected. Eileen Shamy comments:[7]

> Sometimes people hearing of our communion services will contest the whole thing on the grounds that the residents will not know what they are doing. Those who have witnessed and participated in these services would refute that. Very wonderful things happen. One day a most refined and well-spoken woman received the bread and wine very reverently and then burst out enthusiastically, 'Boy, that was good!'

As long ago as 1981, Martha Brown and James Ellor[20] stated the view that feelings remain intact and appropriate in people with Alzheimer's disease.[9] For those with faith in a personal relationship with their God, surely it is arrogant to assume that they have been forgotten as well as forgetting so much themselves. Many people feel forgotten by their own faith communities (see Case Study 15.4).

Case Study 15.4

A Jewish patient was supported by the psychiatric team for the elderly. He had been an elder in the synagogue and the life of their religious community had been very important to him and his wife. They were distressed and lonely because none of the congregation of the synagogue ever visited them once he was unable to attend the synagogue himself because of his dementia.

Person-centred care and spiritual needs

People have different personalities, needs, interests, preferences and, above all, different feelings about themselves and the world around them. Different types of dementing illnesses react with different personalities to produce unique situations. No one solution or set of rules will be right for everyone. Person-centred care focuses on the individual. Iain McGregor and Janet Bell[21] challenged the widely held beliefs that people with dementia cannot make choices, that they wander aimlessly and lose their ability for new learning. They point out that a well-designed environment can minimise dangers and thus allow residents to make decisions for themselves about how they spend their day. They acknowledge that this may be impossibly exhausting for a carer on their own, but in a specialist unit the result is a dynamic community with much interaction and group control.

Aimless wandering can be another misperceived expectation of those caring for those with advanced dementia. I once heard a very moving story about wandering that was misinterpreted with near disastrous results (see Case Study 15.5). Another patient of my own was apparently aggressive with an elderly lady, but again his actions were misinterpreted (see Case Study 15.6).

Case Study 15.5

A man lived in a residential home. He was noticed by the night staff to wander at night. Concern was becoming greater when observation revealed that he always went to a particular female resident's room. Discussion followed about the need for sedation or more draconian measures at this 'sexual' behaviour disorder. Fortunately, it was suggested that he was observed in detail first. On several nights he was observed to enter the old lady's room and bend down near to the head of her bed. He looked at her clock, read the time and then returned to his own room. A clock with a clear dial on his own bedside precluded the need for any more drastic measures.

Case Study 15.6

A man with advanced dementia was nursed in a special hospital unit for those with challenging behaviour. At the time of the Gulf War when much gunfire and bombing featured on the national news, he started trying to escape from the unit, dragging a female patient with him. With patience it was established that he was convinced the building was under fire and he was trying to escape, rescuing the lady with him.

An appreciation of the individual, their life experience and identity can help in all aspects of care, particularly for those with dementia.

Conclusions

Spirituality can be defined in many ways. I like the following:

> Spirituality can be described as a search for that which gives meaning and identity to a person's life and the wider world. Dementia does not destroy the ability to experience and appreciate the world about the person.

This is well illustrated by Paul Wilson writing in *Spirituality and Ageing*,[22] which illustrates several of the points made in this chapter (see Case Study 15.7).

Case Study 15.7

Paul Wilson describes a sequence of events on a visit.
    The door opened and I was greeted by Alan and Barbara (the names are pseudonyms). Alan took me through the kitchen and stopped at his wife's activity table. On it were simple jigsaws, crayons, paper and materials. Alan told me how Barbara spent an hour or so at a time at the table. He celebrated all she could do. As we spoke, a video of Pavarotti was playing in the lounge. We stood and watched as Barbara joyfully danced, totally unaware of, or inhibited by, our presence. Alan spoke of her love of music and the enjoyment she received from the video, dancing and singing along to it. He expressed the hope that one day she would play the piano again. We sat down in the lounge and Barbara, the homemaker, went around all the pictures in the room, telling me about each one in great detail, but unfortunately her speech was jumbled. Barbara has dementia.

I feel I can do no better than sum up the message of this chapter in Paul Wilson's words:

> Care giving is thus more than the provision of a safe environment and communication with others; it is also the provision of spiritual care to nurture the person in the journey within and pastoral care to nurture the person in the journey above.

He quotes Buckland,[23] who talks of the 'fragile web of well-being' which is made up of strands of strength and positive experience. A living environment needs to take into account the effects that change and the ageing process are having on the person. Their values are developed in the core of their being by interacting with their experience and environment over the whole of their life. These values must be built into care giving so that the person does not find themselves in an environment foreign to their lifestyle. We must remember that the person, however hidden from us by the fog of dementia, is still there and can still appreciate their surroundings. As Alison Froggatt so tellingly puts it in her book with Eileen Shamy:[6]

> The sacrament of the present moment has particular poignancy in dementia, for most happenings may be forgotten soon afterwards. But the rose smells just as sweet *now*, and the birds on the bird table are squabbling *now*, and we can laugh.

Above all, we should learn to love those we care for. As Peter Huxham[24] points out, relationships are the only things which change people. We accept that principle in the care of children, but it applies throughout life. As the children's story quoted by Huxham so tellingly illustrates, loving relationships are essential to well-being:[25]

> 'What is real' asked the Rabbit one day, when they were lying side by side near the nursery fender, because Nana came to tidy the room. 'Does it mean having things that buzz inside you and a stick-out handle?'
> 'Real isn't how you are made,' said the Skin Horse. 'It's a thing that happens to you. When a child loves you for a long, long time, not just to play with but *really* loves you, then you become real.'
> (From *The Velveteen Rabbit* by Margery Williams)

Spiritual aspects of dementia include the meeting of spiritual needs, but it is also essential to recognise the need in all humans for a 'sacred space' and the help needed to preserve or recreate such a space. A friend recently talked about her adjustment to retirement, including the adjustment to less 'doing' and more time for 'being'. Laraine Moffitt[26] compares religion as the 'doing' and spirituality as the 'being'. She suggests that learning to attend to someone's spiritual needs requires a shift of emphasis from helping them to *do* something, to providing the environment to allow them to *be*.

Key points

- Spirituality is the search for the meaning of life; religion is one way of conducting the search.
- Spiritual needs can be attended to by truly individualised care.
- Persons with dementia are indeed persons with emotions and feelings.
- Person-centred care is essential for well-being, especially in dementia care.
- Much current writing and legislation on dementia care does not take account of the spiritual dimension of person-centred care.
- Advanced dementia does not preclude enjoyment, loving relationships or creativity.
- People who are members of a faith community need to have continuing contact and will benefit from participation in faith practice.

References

1   Swinton J (2001) *Spirituality and Mental Health Care.* Jessica Kingsley, London.
2   Krishna Mohan K (2001) Spirituality and well-being: an overview. In: M Cornelissen (ed.) *Consciousness and its Transformation.* Sri Aurobindo Ashram Press, Pondicherry.
3   Stoter D (1995) *Spiritual Aspects of Health Care.* Mosby, London.
4   Kitwood T (1997) *Dementia Reconsidered.* Open University Press, Buckingham.
5   Froggatt A (1988) Self-awareness in early dementia. In: B Gearing, M Johnson and T Heller (eds) *Mental Health Problems in Old Age.* Open University Press, Buckingham.
6   Froggatt A and Shamy E (1998) *Dementia: a christian perspective.* Christian Council on Ageing Publications, Derby.
7   Shamy E (1997) *More than Body, Brain and Breath.* ColCom Press, New Zealand. (Edited version by Albert Jewell (2003) under title *A Guide to the Spiritual Dimension of Care for People with Alzheimer's Disease and Related Dementia.* Jessica Kingsley, London.)
8   Kitwood T (1995) Cultures of care: tradition and change. In: T Kitwood and S Benson (eds) *The New Culture of Dementia Care.* Hawker Publications, London.
9   Goldsmith M (1996) *Hearing the Voice of People with Dementia.* Jessica Kingsley, London.
10   Killick J (ed.) (1997) *You are Words.* Hawker Publications, London.
11   Killick J and Cordonnier C (eds) *Openings.* Hawker Publications, London.
12   HMSO (2003) *Care Homes for Older People: National Minimum Standards* (3e). HMSO, London.
13   Alzheimer's Society (2001) Quality Dementia Care in Care Homes: Person-Centred Stanards. AS, London.
14   Johnson AM and Hickman Morris H (2000) *Understanding the Needs of Older People.* Leveson Centre, Paper 1.

15   ONS (1996) *Living in Britain: results from the General Household Survey 1994.* HMSO, London.
16   Crossley D (1995) Religious experience within mental illness. *British Journal of Psychiatry.* **166**: 284–6.
17   Sims ACP (1994) 'Psyche': spirit as well as mind? *British Journal of Psychiatry.* **165**: 441–6.
18   Peck SM (1993) *Further Along the Road Less Travelled.* Simon and Schuster, London.
19   Hammond G and Moffitt L (2000) *Guidelines for Care Plans.* Christian Council on Ageing Publications, Derby and Faith in Elderly People, Leeds.
20   Brown M and Ellor J (1981) An approach to the treatment of symptoms caused by cognitive disorders in the aged. *Salud Publications:* **23**. Cincinatti, OH.
21   McGregor I and Bell J (1994) Buzzing with life, energy and drive. *Journal of Dementia Care.* **1**(6): 20–1.
22   Wilson P (1999) Memory, personhood and faith. In: A Jewell (ed.) *Spirituality and Ageing.* Jessica Kingsley, London.
23   Buckland S (1995) Well-being, personality and residential care. In: T Kitwood and S Benson (eds) *The New Culture of Dementia Care.* Hawker Publications, London.
24   Huxham P (2000) 'I'm not very religious, but …'. In: G Corley (ed.) *Older People and Their Needs.* Whurr Publishers, London.
25   Williams M (1922) *The Velveteen Rabbit.* Heinemann, London.
26   Moffitt L (1996) Helping to recreate a personal sacred space. *Journal of Dementia Care.* **4**(3): 19–21.

Further reading

Regan D and Smith J (1997) *The Fullness of Time.* Counsel and Care, London.
Post SG (1995) *The Moral Challenge of Alzheimer Disease.* Johns Hopkins University Press, Baltimore, MD.
Kitwood T, Buckland S and Petre T (1995) *Brighter Futures.* Anchor Housing Association, Oxford.
Koenig HG (1994) *Ageing and God: spiritual pathways to mental health in mid-life and later years.* Haworth Pastoral Press, New York.
Christian Council on Ageing (2002) *Religious Practice and People with Dementia: a resource for carers.* Edited by Reverend B Allen. CCOA Publications, Derby.
Orchard H (ed.) (2001) *Spirituality in Health Care Contexts.* Jessica Kingsley, London.

16

Developing a comprehensive and integrated mental health service for people with dementia

Ann McPherson

Although the world is very full of suffering, it is also full of the overcoming of it.

(Helen Keller)

Introduction

We are on a journey to create fully integrated health and social care services, for older people that support positive mental health. Approximately 600 000 people in the UK have dementia; this represents 5% of the total population aged 65, rising to 20% of the population aged 80. There are also 17 000 people in younger age groups with dementia in the UK. A staggering 154 000 people with dementia live alone. It is estimated that by 2026 there will be 840 000 people with dementia in the UK, rising to 1.2 million by 2050.

The National Service Framework for Older People,[1] which was published in March 2001, identified in Standard 7 the expectations for services in relation to the mental health needs of older people. It stated: 'Older people who have mental health problems should have access to integrated mental health services, provided by the National Health Service and local authorities, to ensure effective diagnosis, treatment and support for them and for their carers'.

Our journey seeks to explore what an integrated service is. Who should be involved in the delivery and what will be the benefits of an integrated service? It also describes a change management approach to implementation which has been found successful and suggests a way forward.

What is an integrated service?

The NSF for Older People asserts that mental health services for older people should be community orientated and provide seamless packages of care and support for older people and their carers. The aspiration for new services is that they should be comprehensive, multidisciplinary, accessible, responsive, individualised, accountable and systematic.

The NSF also encourages investment in preventive strategies and improving access to specialist care. One of the key challenges it poses is to provide early recognition and management of mental health problems in primary care, supported by specialist old age mental health teams. One of the key milestones clearly stated within the NSF is that by April 2004, Health Investment Plans and other relevant local plans should have included the development of an integrated mental health service for older people that is inclusive of mental health promotion.

This is not dissimilar to the approach adopted by the Health Advisory Service, who, in the document *Standards for Mental Health Services for Older People*,[2] suggest that 'there is a comprehensive specialist mental health service, provided within agreed service criteria, which aims to maintain people at home where possible and preferable'.

The Audit Commission[3] found that the majority of older people preferred to be cared for in their own homes. Other recent studies have also shown that the use of community-based services is preferable to hospital inpatient services for many hospital-eligible clients. The Audit Commission suggests that this balance should be effected through the development of community mental health teams, who can undertake a large part of the assessment and treatment of older people with mental health problems. Its national study showed that those areas which had effective community mental health teams enabled older people to remain at home for longer periods of time.

Who should be involved in providing an integrated service?

The Audit Commission reports[3,4] suggest that sources of referral to mental health services for older people could be from GPs, residential care, social care, nursing homes, advocacy services, acute hospitals, carers and service users themselves.

The philosophy that underpins the service should be the principle that each person is an individual. This is reflected in Standard 2 of the NSF ('Person-centred Care'). As such, individuals have a right to the highest standard of professional, person-centred practice that maintains the dignity, identity and independence of individual clients and so promotes the quality of their life. The objective is to provide a partnership in medical, nursing and therapy expertise, in order to provide a seamless care pathway covering the comprehensive spectrum of care from assessment, treatment, rehabilitation, community mental health nursing, respite care, day services and continuing care. However, in order for it to be truly comprehensive, it needs to encompass the skills and expertise of staff both within housing and social care as well as the voluntary and independent sectors. The pathway also needs to support a shared understanding of, and respect for, individuals' roles and responsibilities, as well as their expectations, underpinned by clear systems for communication, negotiation and decision making.

Why have an integrated service?

The National Beds Inquiry[5] reports that as many as 29% of admissions to acute mental health beds would not have been necessary had resources been available to provide care at home or within a community setting. The Audit Commission found that at least 50% of the assessment process could have been undertaken at home if the appropriate balance of services had been in place. As previously mentioned, it also highlighted that assessments undertaken at home were found to be far more effective.

The Audit Commission states[4] that when developing services for older people with a mental health problem that offer fast and convenient treatment, the range and balance of these require consideration. This is necessary because reconfiguration to improve the range and balance should also increase access to the service. The Audit Commission proposes that accepting referrals from a wide range of sources can also increase accessibility to a service. What it also suggests is that this enables the service to be far more responsive.

There is growing evidence to suggest that providing a comprehensive range of high-quality services that are delivered as close to home as possible and that focus upon enablement, is a key factor in preventing unnecessary admission to hospital, nursing or residential care.

The Audit Commission report 'Forget Me Not 2002'[4] quite clearly identifies that true integration of health and social care services provides for a system of support that is not only seamless but also efficient and effective.

The strategies highlighted within these key documents seek to empower and enhance the lives of service users and their carers, providing them with knowledge, understanding and opportunities to participate in stimulating activities in order that they can make informed decisions and enjoy a meaningful life by:

- rooting out age discrimination
- providing person-centred care
- promoting older people's health and independence
- fitting services around people's needs.

Also clearly evident is that real involvement of users of the services, those who care for them and/or their advocates is fundamental to the commissioning, development and management of services as well as to the delivery of their individual care.

The National Carers Strategy[6] states that local carers groups should have ongoing contact and involvement with local service provisions. The Audit Commission[4] found that carers need information and training. It went on to suggest that the benefits of such schemes, which are designed to give them information and training, are as follows:

- they increase knowledge
- they reduce stress

- they reduce perceived unmet needs for resources (without necessarily increasing the use of resources)
- they delay admissions into residential care.

Developing an integrated service

The task of drawing services together can seem daunting, especially when a wide range of professions and, indeed, employers are involved. It can be difficult to know where to start. However, if a systematic approach is used, the whole thing becomes much more straightforward. One such approach is the RAID model (see Box 16.1), which has been widely introduced to the NHS through the work of the NHS Clinical Governance Support Team. The development of a shared vision, supported by 'values and principles', is only the beginning. Clarity is required on who should be involved in planning and providing integrated mental health services.

Box 16.1　The RAID Model

The RAID model – a systematic approach:

- REVIEW – take a fresh look
- AGREE – engage people in making things better
- IMPLEMENT – make things better
- DEMONSTRATE – patients benefit.

A stakeholder event was organised for the key players in the commissioning and prioritisation of mental health services for older people. During the session, they explored the values and principles that they believed should underpin an integrated service. They reached consensus on a definition of an integrated service. They also achieved a shared vision of the key processes that could support such a service. By the end of the session, they had arrived at a strategy that would provide the framework for delivering an integrated service for older people that is a requirement of the NSF for Older People. As well as a shared vision, they had also created shared enthusiasm, and the potential to implement changes with optimism and genuine partnership.

Review

This involves the following:

- taking a fresh look at the current situation and preparing for change
- involving key stakeholders and understanding their agendas
- identifying the levers that will assist in achieving change

- undertaking a formal review of current practice
- undertaking a literature review of 'best practice'
- gaining support from senior managers
- undertaking interviews with key staff
- holding focus groups not only with groups of staff within the service but also with users of the service and their carers.

Holding focus groups is one of the key processes for getting people on board with the changes that will take services forward. They provide an opportunity for people to look at the things that they consider are done well, and also the things that could be done better. They allow for the exploration of areas which would lead to improvements within the service, and also areas of interest that people might have that could lead to positive change. It identifies people who are enthusiastic, energetic and willing to be involved and provide leadership for the projects to improve services.

Agree

This needs to ensure that people are signed up to change. This part of the model is about understanding who the people are that need to be involved and the 'what's in it for me' agenda. What might people stand to lose or win from the changes that will be implemented? What actions might be required? It is very important at this stage to ensure that you have achieved a shared vision and values underpinned by clarity and ownership about core values. A further key factor is to acknowledge the barriers to change (see Box 16.2).

Box 16.2   Overcoming barriers to change

A useful approach in overcoming barriers to change has been the Protected Time Programme introduced through the NHS Clinical Governance Support Team to develop ways to ensure front-line clinical staff can be released to spend time on service development.

There are a number of barriers to be overcome in moving towards truly integrated services. Often staff of any discipline will cite time as being the key factor in being able to make and sustain change. Often attitudes, values and beliefs, which are legacies of the past, compound this. Another common factor is staff turnover, not helped by the inability to recruit to vacant posts. A lack of long-term planning can contribute to the demotivation and disenchantment of staff, often resulting in services working at full capacity and therefore unable to respond by providing rapid access to some parts of the service. A significant barrier can be the bureaucracy within services, which inhibits the creativity of staff who feel dis-empowered by the hierarchies that exist. One of the most important things that can help to smooth the way is gaining executive-level commitment to the work to be undertaken. This helps to ensure the momentum by keeping things on track.

Implement

This needs to make things better. In undertaking this part of the model, it is important to select projects that put patients at the centre and will improve the process of care. They need to be in line with organisational priorities and need to demonstrate that there is strong clinical leadership and that there is ownership at a local level. This can be achieved by selecting people whose leadership potential can be developed by undertaking selected projects.

When putting the proposed changes into place, thought should be given to keeping the rules simple, ensuring that multiple small experiments are undertaken and that monitoring of the work is ongoing. It is also important to recognise that the work will cover a range of projects, from ones that are long term through to medium term, in relation to implementation, but that most importantly it is necessary to ensure that quick wins are included, as these will:

- show rapid results

- build energy and momentum

- gain confidence in implementing change.

Demonstrate

Do patients benefit? What are the things that have been achieved by the projects? Have we done the things that we said we would do? Have we improved the service for the patients? Clinical governance is about building partnerships with patients to ensure that we continuously strive to improve the quality of care that we deliver, and that we do so in a way that is systematic and accountable (see Box 16.3).

Box 16.3   Building partnerships with patients

Quick win – patients in an assessment unit were dependent on nursing staff to provide their breakfasts. Often nursing staff were busy, which resulted in delays to the time patients could expect breakfast. Breakfast bars and drinks facilities were introduced to the unit and patients were able to help themselves. Both patients and staff evaluated this initiative extremely positively.

One year after service changes were introduced, the Older People's Mental Health Service staff focus group was repeated. Staff felt that they were:

- delivering quality, person-centred care
- increasing their critical awareness of practice
- good at responding to challenges
- good at learning from experiences.

Overall they felt that the service was very adaptable and flexible around the needs of patients, and that there was a culture developing that embraced change rather than tried to avoid it.

Having demonstrated that the changes put in place have achieved genuine improvements, it is then time to move back to the review stage and start all over again.

Key successes

True engagement of people who use services, their carers, and health professionals from primary care, acute hospitals, mental health services, local authorities, and the independent and voluntary sector are necessary to secure and develop a 'shared vision' for the way forward. This has to be supported by values and principles, which underpin the delivery of integrated services, thereby providing integrated care.

The focus has to be on ensuring person-centred care that:

- is easily accessible, ensuring assessment and treatment are timely
- is needs led, not service driven
- involves individuals and their carers in decisions about the care required, which will respect their choices, their opinions and the ability to support their personal freedom whilst ensuring effective risk assessment and management
- empowers individuals so that they feel able to criticise as well as praise
- ensures individuals and their carers are listened to and treated with respect, confidentiality and honesty and that their privacy and dignity is maintained at all times
- respects individuals and their carers' spiritual and cultural needs.

Improving the care of older people with dementia depends on providing high-quality, evidence-based care. It is also dependent on their carers receiving information, advice and practical help to support them in caring. Early diagnosis gives access to treatment, allows for the planning of future care, and helps individuals and their carers to come to terms with their progress.

The provision of a responsive and comprehensive range of high-quality, flexible mental health services for the older person and people with dementia should be delivered through a person-centred approach which is clearly understood.

Additionally, a number of key processes are also necessary to support the delivery of such services. Examples include:

- single point of access

- single integrated documentation system

- single assessment process that includes risk assessment and is underpinned by integrated assessment and care management/care programme approach (CPA)

- health promotion and shared protocols for the early detection of mental health problems within older people

- performance indicators and review processes.

Indicators of success

According to Ellis and Whittington,[7] quality within healthcare is being able to demonstrate that standards are maintained and resources are used as effectively as possible. Therefore success would be demonstrated by a much better, speedier journey through the service for individuals. They should be able to expect:

- improved outcomes in their care

- improved satisfaction with the service

- less dependence on the services

- increased quality of life

- increased confidence in the service by both them and their carers.

Indicators of success are important both for service users and professional staff. At a local stakeholder event, organised to look at mental health services for older people, the following were identified as indicators of success that would improve the journey for the patient:

- shorter waiting lists

- reduction in the number of beds blocked

- better use of resources

- improved staff satisfaction

- individuals' time used more appropriately – service users and service providers

- reduction in admissions to hospital with emergencies managed more effectively in the community

- individuals receiving care that is responsive to their needs

- reduction in duplication of services by different agencies
- accurate identification of gaps within services.

Rigorous performance monitoring and evaluation of current and future service provision and its outcomes are essential if this journey is to continue.

Suggestions for the future

Clearly, in looking to the future, services should wherever possible focus on maintaining care for the individual at home. To be able to do this, it is essential that an individual's care needs are co-ordinated by one person (usually the Care Co-ordinator), and that they know who to talk to not only about their care but also who to contact in a crisis.

Services also need to be able to provide specialist input, ensuring that care delivery involves the right person with the right skills at the right time. They need to ensure that the skills of the staff are utilised effectively and appropriately, and therefore their input is recognised and their professional opinions are respected.

Services need to take up the challenge of being innovative, constantly striving to improve and develop new models of care in response to people's needs. Greater use of Health Act Flexibilities, which allow for the pooling of budgets by health and social services, will support innovative approaches to the delivery of care.

Services have to continue to expand their work with carers, supporting them and applying their values and principles, in order to develop genuinely trusting relationships between service users, providers of care and commissioners of care. This should ensure that services are effectively co-ordinated and maintain a transparent approach.

A shared understanding of services has to be agreed by all key stakeholders in order for there to be flexibility across agencies and strong interagency links. They must use the same language and share the same expectations.

Key points

- The involvement of service users, carers and front-line staff is the key to success for developing integrated services.
- The support of the executive management team provides strategic impact – opens doors and keeps implementation on track.
- It is important that the work people undertake is an integral part of their role.
- Action is a key word focusing on what can be achieved.
- Celebrate success and give people the recognition for work well done – it builds momentum and sustains change.

The journey towards a society where older people are no longer seen as a burden continues. They are a vital source of wisdom, experience and talent.

References

1   Department of Health (2001) *National Service Framework for Older People.* DoH, London.
2   Health Advisory Service (2000) *Standards for Mental Health Services for Older People.* Pavilion Publishing, Brighton.
3   Audit Commission (2000) *Forget Me Not: mental health services for older people.* Audit Commission, London.
4   The Audit Commission Update (2002) *Forget Me Not 2002.* Audit Commission, London.
5   Department of Health (2000) *Shaping the Future NHS: long-term planning for hospital and related services.* Consultation document on the findings of the National Bed Inquiry. DoH, London.
6   Department of Health (1999) *Caring about Carers: a national strategy for carers.* HMSO, London.
7   Ellis R and Whittington D (1993) *Quality Assurance in Health Care: a handbook.* Edward Arnold, London.

Conclusion

We hope you have enjoyed reading this book and that you think we have at least partly achieved a synthesis of a modern, scientific understanding and a thoroughly practical, multidisciplinary approach to meeting the needs of people with dementia. Those planning and providing services for people with dementia need a capacity to work well with other professionals, and with relatives and carers, if they are to achieve satisfaction in their work and the best outcomes for their patients and carers. They also need to constantly update their understanding of the scientific and social background to their practice. They need to understand what is important for patients and carers. A book of this length can never be fully comprehensive, but we hope that it will serve as a ready reference for those working in the field and perhaps inspire them to continue improving the service we offer to this uniquely vulnerable and often neglected group in our society.

Stephen Curran
John Wattis

Index